GET THE F*CK IN SHAPE

A GUIDE FOR THE FITNESSLY-CHALLENGED

BY INDIANA JETHRO BUMSTEAD

INDEX

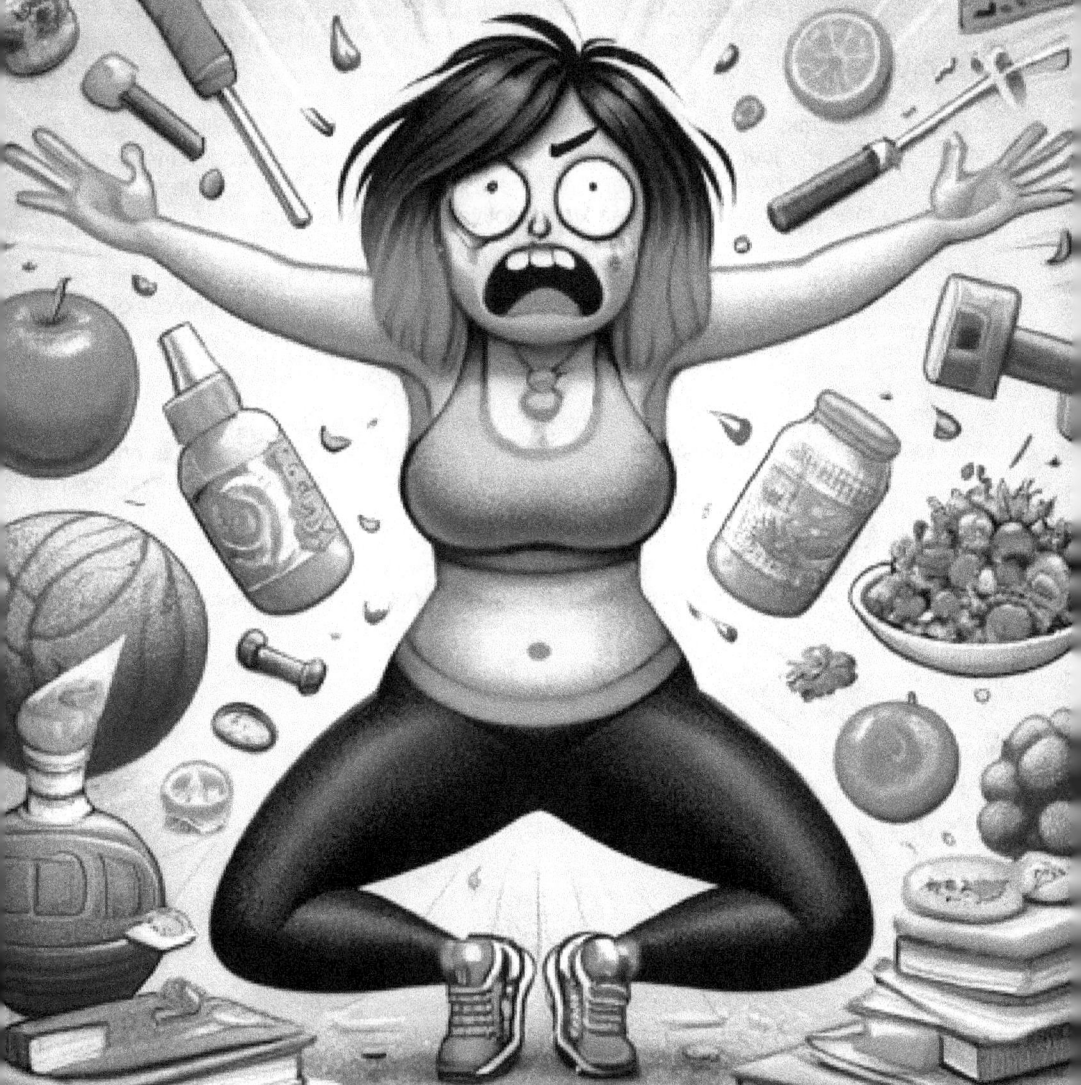

EPIC PREFACE

Greetings, Mortals,

I am Hercules, son of Zeus, known throughout the ages for my legendary strength and twelve labors of mythic proportions. As I gaze down from the lofty heights of Mount Olympus, I have witnessed the valor and struggles of humanity in its quest for health and vitality. It is in this spirit that I lend my voice to the preface of "Get The F*ck In Shape : A Guide for the Fitnessly-Challenged" by Indiana Jethro Bumstead.

In my time, the pursuit of physical excellence was a matter of honor and necessity, often entwined with the whims of gods and the fates of kingdoms. However, in this modern era, the quest for fitness has taken on a different hue. It is a battle not against mythical beasts or vengeful gods, but against the more insidious foes of lethargy, routine, and the siren call of the couch.

Indiana Jethro Bumstead, in his unique tome, presents an odyssey not unlike the labors I once undertook. His journey from a sedentary mortal to one who embraces the vigor of physical exertion is both inspiring and, I daresay, entertaining. Through his words, he conjures laughter as a balm for the weary and motivation for the hesitant.

Yet, let it be known that the path to Herculean strength and Olympian fitness does not require divine intervention or feats of legend. Instead, it is found in the daily choices of each mortal - the decision to rise, to move, to challenge oneself, and to find joy in the journey towards health.

As you embark upon this literary journey with Indiana, remember that the strength of Hercules lies not solely in muscle and sinew, but in the heart and determination of one who faces their challenges head-on. May you find within these pages the spark to ignite your own journey, to transform not just in body, but in spirit.

Embrace your labors with the mirth of Dionysus and the resolve of Athena. And fear not the road ahead, for within each of you lies the potential for greatness, the heart of a hero, and the spirit of a god.

In Strength and Laughter,

Hercules, Son of Zeus,
Mount Olympus.

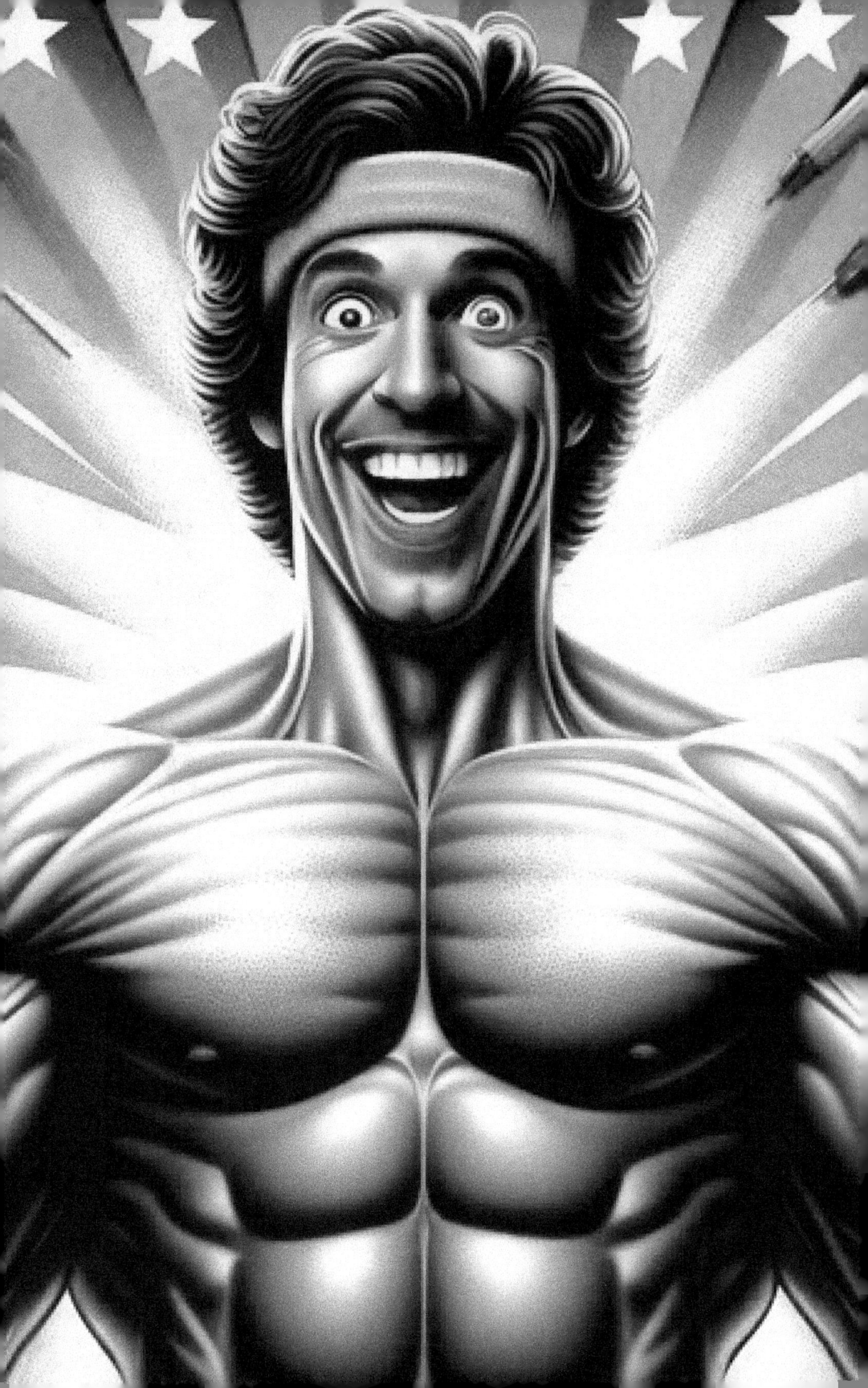

OFFICIAL PREFACE

As a physician dedicated to the well-being of my patients, I am often asked about the best ways to achieve and maintain good health. Time and again, my advice centers on two fundamental principles: balanced nutrition and regular physical activity. When Indiana Jethro Bumstead approached me to pen a preface for his book, "Get The F*ck In Shape : A Guide for the Fitnessly-Challenged," I was intrigued. After delving into its pages, I found it to be a refreshing, humorous, and surprisingly insightful take on the often daunting world of fitness and health.

In a society where health advice is frequently delivered in a manner that's either overly clinical or dauntingly prescriptive, Indy's book stands out as a beacon of hope and humor. It reminds us that the journey to health doesn't have to be a solemn or tedious affair; it can be filled with laughter, self-discovery, and an abundance of joy.

As a doctor, I have seen firsthand how a positive mindset can significantly impact one's health journey. Indy's anecdotes and advice, although delivered with a generous dose of humor, encapsulate this principle beautifully. He encourages readers to embrace fitness not as a chore, but as a delightful part of life, an approach I wholeheartedly endorse.

However, it is important to remember, as Indy himself points out, that this book is not a substitute for professional medical advice. It is a companion to motivate and inspire you on your health journey. As you navigate the path to better health, I encourage you to consult with healthcare professionals to create a plan that is tailored to your individual needs.

"Get The F*ck In Shape" is a reminder that health and happiness are intrinsically linked. Indy's transformation from a fitness-phobic to a fitness enthusiast is not just about physical changes. It's a story of how altering one's lifestyle and perspective can lead to a richer, more fulfilling life.

Whether you are taking your first tentative steps towards a healthier lifestyle or looking for a way to add joy to your existing health routine, this book is a wonderful resource. It offers laughter as a form of medicine and positivity as a tool for change. I hope that as you turn these pages, you find not only entertainment but also inspiration to make health and fitness an enjoyable and integral part of your life.

Sincerely,

Dr. Jane H. Goodwell, M.D

EDITOR'S NOTE

Dear Soon-to-be-Fitter and Happier Reader,

If you're holding this book and wondering if it's going to be yet another preachy tome that makes you feel guilty about skipping leg day, rest easy. This is not that book. As the proud yet slightly bewildered editor of Indiana Jethro Bumstead's hilariously honest journey from a donut-devouring couch potato to a somewhat less donut-devouring fitness enthusiast, I'm here to give you a foreword that's as heartfelt as it is light-hearted.

Firstly, a confession: When Indy first brought his manuscript to us, half the office ended up in fits of laughter, and the other half in bewildered shock at how someone could be so disarmingly honest about their struggles with fitness. We knew right then that we had a book that was going to make waves – mostly from readers falling over in laughter.

Indy's journey is one that many of us can relate to. It's not about transforming into a model on a fitness magazine cover. It's about the real, sometimes messy and often funny journey towards getting in shape, or at least, towards not getting winded while climbing a flight of stairs.

Throughout this book, you'll find stories that might feel a little too familiar. Like the time Indy got locked into a somewhat compromising position in a yoga class and had to be rescued by an amused instructor. Or his first encounter with a salad that contained more leaves than an autumn yard (his words, not mine). These stories are told with such humor and candor that you can't help but nod along, thinking, "Yep, been there, done that." But it's not just about the laughs (though there are plenty). Indy's journey is a testament to the fact that fitness is accessible to everyone. You don't need to be a natural athlete or have a gym membership since the dawn of time. All you need is a bit of determination, a willingness to laugh at yourself, and perhaps a good pair of sneakers.

So, as you turn these pages and embark on this journey with Indy, remember: fitness is a personal journey, and it's okay to take it one step (or one chuckle) at a time. Prepare to be entertained, inspired, and perhaps a little motivated to start your own journey.

Enjoy the ride, and remember – if you're reading this while training, watch out for low-hanging branches or street poles. We're not responsible for any reading-induced hazards!

Marina C. Lovedar
Editor-in-Chief, Extra-Extra Publishi

AUTHOR'S FOREWORD

Dear Reader (or accidental book-picker-upper),

If you're expecting a tale of an overnight transformation from couch potato to fitness model, let me set the record straight: this is not that story. In fact, when I first started my journey to Get The F*ck In Shape, my idea of a hardcore workout was reaching across the couch to grab the remote – and if I really wanted to push the envelope, I'd reach for the snacks on the coffee table.

I'm Indiana Jethro Bumstead, but you can call me Indy, and this is my not-so-heroic tale of going from "I think my sofa is eating me" to "Hey, I can see my toes again!" It's a story filled with sweat, the occasional tear (mostly from laughter), and the kind of exercise routines that wouldn't scare off a sloth.

I should confess – when I first thought about getting fit, I imagined it would be like in the movies. There'd be this epic montage where I'd be lifting weights in slow motion, running along beaches, and at the end of a three-minute power ballad, I'd emerge transformed. The reality? I discovered that my running style is less 'graceful gazelle' and more 'newborn giraffe on roller skates.'

This book is my journey, but it's also a collection of the hilariously painful truths I learned about getting in shape. Like how doing a push-up for the first time in years can feel like trying to lift a small car. Or that yoga isn't just "fancy stretching" – it's a crafty form of gymnastics designed by people who clearly don't have bones.

But amidst all the huffing, puffing, and giggling at myself in the mirror, I found something unexpected – a sense of joy and accomplishment in taking care of my body. I learned that fitness isn't just about how you look; it's about how you feel, how you laugh, and how you live.

So, whether you're a gym junkie or someone who considers walking to the fridge a decent trek, I invite you to join me on this clumsy, comical, and maybe even inspiring journey to better health. Let's face it, if I can do it, anyone can. And who knows? You might even have a bit of fun along the way.

Here's to the misfits, the late bloomers, and everyone who's ever thought, "Maybe tomorrow I'll start exercising." Our time is now – or, you know, after the next chapter.

In Sweat and Laughter,

Indiana Jethro Bumstead, aspiring author and life-coach.

PROLOGUE

If you had told me a few years ago that I would be writing a book about fitness, I would have laughed so hard I might have actually burned a calorie or two. Hi, I'm Indiana Jethro Bumstead, but you can call me Indy, and this is the story of how a certified couch potato turned into, well, a slightly more active potato with a newfound love for fitness.

I was the guy who thought 'cardio' was a type of cheese and 'burpees' were just unfortunate bodily functions. The closest I came to a marathon was binge-watching TV shows while marathoning through a family-sized bag of chips. My idea of heavy lifting involved hoisting a large pizza all the way from the delivery box to my mouth. But, as fate would have it, I embarked on a fitness journey that was as unplanned as it was transformative. It started with a pair of jeans - my favorite pair - that decided one day they were no longer going to fit. After a grueling battle, which involved a lot of huffing, puffing, and muttered expletives, I had to accept defeat. It was the wake-up call I didn't know I needed. Stepping into a gym for the first time was like walking onto another planet. A planet where gravity seemed to have increased tenfold and where every piece of equipment looked like a torture device from medieval times. I was the awkward new kid, fumbling around and trying to look like I knew what I was doing while secretly fearing for my life.

I won't lie; the initial phase of my fitness journey was about as graceful as a hippo on ice skates. There were mishaps - oh, so many mishaps. Like the time I confidently stepped onto a treadmill, not realizing it was already running, and got ejected off the back with the grace of a rag doll. Or when I attempted to lift weights that were clearly out of my league and almost became a sad headline in the local news. Despite the bumpy start, something miraculous happened. I started to enjoy the process. I began to look forward to the gym, to the workouts, and even to the sore muscles that reminded me I was getting stronger. I discovered the joys of endorphins, those magical little hormones that make you feel like maybe, just maybe, you're a superhero in training.

This book is more than just my journey from fitness phobic to fitness fanatic. It's a collection of stories, tips, and a whole lot of humor about getting into shape. It's for anyone who's ever felt out of place in a gym, for anyone who's thought that 'running' is just something your nose does in the winter, and for anyone who's looking for a laugh while they embark on their fitness journey. So, buckle up, grab your favorite snack (because let's be real, old habits die hard), and get ready to embark on a journey filled with humor, self-discovery, and maybe, just a little bit of sweating. Welcome to the world of fitness according to Indiana Jethro Bumstead - where the laughs are plentiful, the workouts are bearable, and the journey is just as important as the destination.

CHAPTER 1.
GETTING "BACK" IN SHAPE

"Fitness is like a relationship. You can't cheat and expect it to work."

I've never been one for fairy tales, but if there's one I'd tell, it would be about the Great Fitness Hoax. This is not the story of a dashing knight conquering dragon-laden workouts or a damsel effortlessly dropping dress sizes. No, this is the tale of an average Joe, yours truly, who thought the most exercise he'd ever get was changing TV channels.

My journey begins not with a bang, but with a whimper—a whimper heard as I tried, and failed, to touch my toes. It's a universal truth, universally ignored, that not everyone was born with a six-pack or the ability to run a marathon. And that's okay. But here I was, staring into the abyss of my bathroom mirror, pondering if the reflection was a cruel joke. The mirror doesn't lie, but oh, how I wished it did.

You see, I come from a long line of what fitness enthusiasts would gently call 'underachievers.' My family's idea of a workout was lifting the remote or, on a good day, walking to the fridge. So, it was no surprise that my first encounter with the gym was less of a heroic undertaking and more of a comedy sketch.

Remember the first time you tried to work out? If you're anything like me, it was less of a Rocky Balboa moment and more like a scene straight out of a sitcom. There I was, a wide-eyed, slightly round individual surrounded by machines that looked like they belonged in a medieval torture chamber. I approached the treadmill with the same enthusiasm one reserves for a dental visit. I had heard myths about these contraptions - they could speed up, incline, and, I suspected, plot my untimely demise.

But let's rewind a bit. Before this foray into the world of sweat and tears, there was the matter of the bathroom scale. Ah, the scale, that little square of doom. It's the one object in your house that can single-handedly determine the course of your day. Step on it and see a number you like, you're walking on sunshine. Step on it and see a number you don't, suddenly it's Adele songs and comfort food. My relationship with my scale was complicated. We were like two arch-nemeses locked in a perpetual dance. Every morning, I'd step on it, and every morning, it seemed to whisper, "I've got your number, buddy." And it did, literally.

This was the catalyst, the moment I realized something had to change. But change is a funny thing; it's like wearing a new pair of underwear. At first, it's uncomfortable, but then it becomes a part of you. I knew I needed to take a self-assessment, but not the kind you'd find in fitness magazines where every answer leads to, "You're perfect, now do some squats!" No, this was going to be a self-assessment sprinkled with a healthy dose of reality and a pinch of sarcasm.

So, I devised my own quiz. Questions like, "How many push-ups can you do? A) What's a push-up? B) Does pushing myself up from the couch count? C) I can do two, and then I cry." It was less about accuracy and more about setting the stage for what was to come. The results were in, and surprise, surprise, I was what the fitness world would call 'a work in progress.'

But every hero's journey has to start somewhere. Mine started at rock bottom, or as I like to call it, the comfortable valley of the couch. I had to face the hard truth that my most significant workout to date was probably the time I spent an entire day binge-watching a TV series. I needed a plan, a workout plan that wouldn't reduce me to tears or leave me feeling like I'd been hit by a bus.

Creating this plan was like drafting a peace treaty between my couch-loving self and this new fitness-warrior persona I was trying to adopt. The key was to keep it simple. I'm talking really simple, like, "Congratulations, you walked around the block without stopping for ice cream" simple. I decided that my fitness journey would be a series of small, almost laughably easy steps. Because let's face it, when you're starting from zero, every step is a victory parade.

And so, armed with nothing but determination and a slightly bruised ego, I embarked on this journey. It was a path littered with challenges, like learning the difference between a burpee and an actual burp (trust me, there's a big one), and facing the dreaded gym for the first time. But it was also a path filled with unexpected joys, like discovering that I could, in fact, run for more than thirty seconds without collapsing.

This, dear reader, is the story of how an average guy, with an average body and an above-average love for pizza, took on the Herculean task of getting in shape. It's a tale of triumphs, setbacks, and the occasional faceplant on a yoga mat. It's the story of how I learned to embrace my inner sloth and become the fitness cheetah I never thought I could be. And if I can do it, so can you.

So buckle up, buttercup. It's going to be a bumpy, hilarious, and, dare I say, inspiring ride.

For starters, let's explore how you can hack your brain to transition from a sedentary lifestyle to aspiring for Olympian-like fitness. It's all about mindset - changing the way you think about exercise and your capabilities. Remember, every great journey begins with a single step, or in this case, a thought.

1. Visualize Your Success:

- Start by visualizing your success. Imagine yourself achieving your fitness goals, whether it's running a marathon, lifting a certain weight, or just feeling more energetic and healthy. Visualization is a powerful tool; it's like setting the GPS for your brain, guiding your actions towards your destination.

2. Set Achievable Goals:
- Set small, achievable goals. Instead of aiming to instantly transform into an Olympian, start with manageable targets. It could be as simple as a 15-minute walk daily or doing ten push-ups every morning. These small goals are your stepping stones, and each one you achieve will build your confidence.

3. The Power of Habit:
- Create a routine. Consistency is key in transforming your mindset. By doing something active at the same time each day, exercise becomes a habit, as natural as brushing your teeth. Your brain starts to expect and even look forward to this regular activity.

4. Positive Affirmations:
- Use positive affirmations to reinforce your commitment. Phrases like "I am getting stronger every day" or "Every step takes me closer to my goal" can be incredibly motivating. Repeat these affirmations daily; they act like cheat codes to boost your mental strength.

5. Educate Yourself:
- Knowledge is power. Read about fitness, watch motivational videos, or listen to health podcasts. The more you know about the benefits of exercise and a healthy lifestyle, the more your brain will be inclined to pursue these goals.

6. Celebrate the Small Victories:
- Every time you choose to exercise instead of sitting on the couch, celebrate it. It could be a mental pat on the back or a small reward like a relaxing bath. These celebrations reinforce positive behavior and make you more likely to repeat it.

7. Find a Workout You Enjoy:
  - Experiment with different types of exercise until you find something you genuinely enjoy. It could be dancing, hiking, swimming, or a sport. When you enjoy what you're doing, it doesn't feel like a chore, and your brain starts to associate exercise with pleasure.

8. Connect with Like-Minded People:
  - Surround yourself with people who have a similar mindset. Join fitness groups, online communities, or workout with a friend. When you're part of a community, motivation and inspiration come more easily.

9. Reflect on Your Progress:
  - Regularly reflect on how far you've come. Keep a journal or simply take time to think about your improvements. This reflection helps your brain recognize and be proud of your progress, fueling further motivation.

10. Be Patient and Kind to Yourself:
  - Lastly, be patient and kind to yourself. Changing a mindset takes time. There will be setbacks, but the key is to keep moving forward. Be your own biggest cheerleader, not your critic.

Remember, transforming from a sedentary lifestyle to that of an Olympian wannabe is as much about mental change as it is about physical change. By hacking your brain with these strategies, you're laying the foundation for a lifetime of health, fitness, and well-being. So start thinking like the athlete you aspire to be, and watch as your body follows suit!

CHAPTER 2.
YOU DON'T NEED TO BE RICH TO BE FIT

"Running: A way to pretend you're a superhero, minus the cape and the ability to fly."

If you've ever wondered what it feels like to be both the hero and the villain in your own story, welcome to your first workout. This is where the true adventure begins, where you bravely step into unknown territory, armed with nothing but a pair of sneakers and a fragile hope that you won't embarrass yourself too badly.

My first workout was a day that will live in infamy. It was the day I realized that the phrase "it's like riding a bike" does not apply to exercise. I had grand illusions of gracefully jogging around the park, maybe doing a few push-ups, and calling it a day. The reality was more akin to a nature documentary where the newborn giraffe tries to walk for the first time.

I chose jogging because, in my mind, it was simple. One foot in front of the other, right? How hard could it be? I had seen people jogging. They always looked so serene, so at peace. Little did I know, jogging is the ultimate act of betrayal. It promises ease and delivers agony.

So there I was, in my brand-new running shoes that were as bright and optimistic as my outlook. I started with a warm-up, which, in retrospect, was more of a 'warm-down.' My stretches were less "flexible yogi" and more "rusty robot." But I was not deterred. I was ready to conquer.

I began my jog with a confidence that was entirely unearned. For the first few minutes, I felt invincible. The wind was in my hair, the sun was on my face, and I was a fitness god. This feeling lasted approximately four minutes. It was around the fifth minute that reality set in, and my body began to ask questions like, "What are we doing?" and "Is this necessary?"

My breathing, which had started as controlled and rhythmic, quickly turned into the desperate gasps of a man who'd just been told there's a shortage of oxygen. My legs, once strong and sure, now felt like they were made of spaghetti - overcooked spaghetti. I was half expecting to hear the Rocky theme music, but all I could hear was the thudding of my heart, which was trying to escape my chest.

But I persevered. I jogged past families in the park who looked at me with a mix of concern and awe. I like to think they were inspired by my determination, but it's more likely they were taking bets on when I'd collapse.

And then it happened. The moment I'd been dreading. The stitch in my side. The stitch, my friends, is nature's way of saying, "Slow down, buddy. Who do you think you are, Usain Bolt?" It's a sharp, stabbing pain that feels like your body is staging a mutiny. I tried to run through it, but it was like trying to ignore a fire alarm.

I slowed to a walk, defeated but not broken. As I walked, I realized something important. Fitness isn't about being the best. It's not about running the fastest or lifting the heaviest. It's about showing up, putting in the effort, and not being too proud to walk when you need to.

That first workout was a disaster by any conventional standard. But it was also a victory. I had taken the first step (and several panting, sweaty steps after that) on my fitness journey. I had faced my fears, battled my body, and lived to tell the tale.

As I limped back home, I knew one thing for sure. This was just the beginning. There would be more workouts, each with its own challenges and triumphs. I was on the path to becoming fitter, stronger, and maybe even a little bit wiser.

So, to anyone standing at the starting line of their fitness journey, I say this: Embrace the awkwardness, the discomfort, and the occasional humiliation. Remember, every athlete was once a beginner. Every marathon runner once struggled to run a mile. You are not alone in your struggle, and there is joy to be found in every painful, hilarious step.

Your first workout is not just a workout. It's a declaration of courage, a testament to your determination. It's the start of a great adventure, one that will take you to places you never thought you could go. And trust me, it's worth every single step.

As we carry on, I'd like to dive into the often-misunderstood concept that getting in shape doesn't necessarily require a hefty financial investment. The notion that fitness is accessible to everyone, regardless of their economic status, is crucial and empowering.

1. The Myth of Costly Fitness: Breaking Down Barriers
- There's a common misconception that staying fit is a luxury only accessible to those with the financial means to pay for gym memberships, personal trainers, and high-end fitness equipment. However, this couldn't be further from the truth. The reality is, fitness is a state of being that you can achieve through various means, many of which cost nothing at all.

2. Bodyweight Exercises: The Free Gym
- Your body itself is a fantastic tool for getting in shape. Bodyweight exercises like push-ups, sit-ups, squats, lunges, and planks require no equipment yet are incredibly effective for building strength and endurance.
- These exercises can be done anywhere – in your living room, a park, or even in a small space like a hotel room. They're like the free apps on your phone – readily available and surprisingly useful.

3. The Great Outdoors: Nature's Playground
- Nature offers a vast, open, and free space for fitness activities. Activities like walking, jogging, hiking, swimming in a lake, or ocean, and cycling on a trail are not only good for your body but also for your soul.
- The outdoors provides a constantly changing environment that can keep your workouts fresh and exciting. It's like having an ever-expanding gym with an infinite number of rooms to explore.

4. Online Resources: A Wealth of Free Information
- The internet is awash with free resources to help you on your fitness journey. From YouTube workout tutorials and fitness blogs to free workout apps and social media fitness communities, there's an abundance of information and guidance available at no cost.
- These resources are akin to having a digital personal trainer and fitness community at your fingertips.

5. Home-Made Equipment: DIY Fitness
- If you prefer working out with equipment, there's no need to break the bank. Common household items can be transformed into workout tools. Cans of food can serve as light weights, a chair can be used for tricep dips, and a towel can be used for resistance exercises.
- This approach not only saves money but also encourages creativity and resourcefulness in your fitness routine.

6. The Power of Consistency: No Cost, High Reward

- Perhaps the most important aspect of fitness is consistency, and that doesn't cost a dime. Sticking to a regular exercise schedule and making healthy dietary choices are key to getting in shape.

- Think of consistency as your daily deposit into your health savings account. Over time, the interest compounds, and the rewards can be enormous.

7. Community Activities: Social Fitness

- Participating in community sports or fitness groups can be a cost-effective way to stay active. Many communities offer free or low-cost fitness classes, group runs, or sports leagues.

- Engaging in these community activities provides the added benefit of social interaction, which can be a powerful motivator.

8. Mindset over Money: The True Wealth of Health

- Ultimately, your mindset is your most valuable asset in getting fit. The belief that you can improve your health regardless of your financial situation is empowering. It's about making the best of what you have and focusing on the wealth of possibilities rather than the limitations.

In conclusion, the path to fitness is as much about ingenuity, determination, and consistency as it is about financial resources. Being broke and fit is absolutely achievable, just as being rich and inactive is a possibility. It all boils down to your choices, your creativity, and your commitment to your health. Remember, the best investment in fitness is your time and effort, and these are resources that everyone possesses.

CHAPTER 3.
PRESS START TO PLAY

"The only bad workout is the one that didn't happen."

Let me tell you a secret about exercise: it's a shapeshifter. It can be anything you want it to be. It can be a vigorous run at dawn, a gentle yoga session at dusk, or, in my case, a series of desperate attempts to move my body in ways that don't induce crying.

After surviving my first workout, which I affectionately call 'The Day of Reckoning,' I realized something crucial: regular exercise doesn't require a gym membership or fancy equipment. It just requires a little creativity and a willingness to look slightly ridiculous in the comfort of your own home.

So, let's embark on this journey of turning mundane daily activities into a fitness fiesta. Here's how I, an average Joe with a penchant for humor and a phobia of gym-timidation, made peace with exercise.

1. The Ninja in the Kitchen: Cooking Calisthenics

Who knew cooking could be a workout? Every time I'm in the kitchen, I see it as an opportunity to tone. Waiting for the pasta to boil? Time for calf raises. Stand on your toes, raise those heels, and feel like a ballerina while you stir that sauce. Your spaghetti might not taste professional, but your calves will look it.

And let's not forget about reaching for those high shelves. Every time I need to grab something from the top shelf, I do a little jump. It's like a mini plyometric workout, and if I'm lucky, I don't knock anything over in the process.

2. The Vacuum Lunge: Household Hygiene with a Twist

Vacuuming: a chore most of us dread. But what if I told you it could be your new favorite workout? Every time I push the vacuum forward, I lunge. Yes, it takes a bit longer to clean the room, but think of the satisfaction. Not only do you end up with a clean carpet, but you also get a mini leg workout. Plus, it's fun to imagine you're lunging away from the dirt, like a hero in an action movie, except the villain is dust bunnies.

3. The Couch Potato Turned Fit Potato

Here's where things get interesting. During every TV commercial break, I set a small goal. Ten sit-ups, fifteen jumping jacks, or just standing up and sitting back down until the show returns. It's surprisingly effective. By the end of an episode, I've done a full workout, and I didn't miss any of the plot twists.

4. The Stairway to Fitness Heaven

Stairs are a gift. Every time I walk past them, I see a challenge. I run up and down a couple of times, pretending I'm training for a dramatic movie role where I'm the underdog turned champion. Sometimes, I take them two at a time to feel like a gazelle, a slightly uncoordinated gazelle, but a gazelle nonetheless.

5. Dance Like No One's Watching (Because They're Not)

This is my favorite. Every day, I have a private dance party. I put on my favorite tunes and just dance around the house. It's liberating, exhilarating, and, most importantly, a great workout. The best part? No one's there to see my questionable dance moves.

Through these humorous yet practical examples, I've found a way to weave exercise into the fabric of my everyday life. It's less about transforming into a fitness model and more about adding a sprinkle of activity here and there. And guess what? It works. Not only do I feel better, but I also find myself looking forward to these quirky little exercise moments.

So, my fellow fitness fledglings, I encourage you to find your unique, perhaps slightly odd, ways to get moving. Remember, exercise doesn't have to be a chore or something you dread. It can be fun, it can be silly, and it can be incredibly rewarding.

After mastering the art of kitchen calisthenics and vacuum lunges, I realized that the world was my oyster—or, more accurately, my personal gym. The possibilities were endless, and my mission to inject a bit of fitness into every nook and cranny of my day became not just a challenge, but a delightful adventure.

6. The Grocery Bag Gauntlet

Grocery shopping is no longer just a mundane task; it's an opportunity for an impromptu workout. I began using my grocery bags as makeshift weights. Carrying them from the car to my kitchen became a test of endurance and strength. Each bag of groceries was a trophy of my triumph over laziness. Walking up the stairs with bags hanging off each arm, I'd imagine myself as a mountaineer, scaling the peaks of Mount Everest, except the peak was my fifth-floor apartment, and my Sherpa was a bag of frozen broccoli.

7. The Secret Agent Walk

Walking is the unsung hero of fitness. I turned my daily walks into a game. Sometimes, I'd pretend to be a secret agent on a mission, taking brisk, purposeful strides. Other times, I'd be a runway model on the catwalk of the sidewalk, strutting my stuff. Each walk became an adventure, a story, a mini escape from the mundane. And the best part? Walking is genuinely good for you. It's low-impact, it's easy, and it can be done almost anywhere.

8. The Laughing Ab Workout

They say laughter is the best medicine, but did you know it's also a workout? I started watching comedy shows and laughing as hard as I could. It might sound silly, but laughing works your abdominal muscles. So, not only was I entertaining myself, but I was also getting a workout. It was multitasking at its finest.

9. The Art of Active Sitting

Sitting down doesn't have to be a passive activity. I began practicing what I call 'active sitting.' While sitting at my desk, I'd do leg raises under the table or clench my glutes. It was like a secret workout, a clandestine operation to strengthen my muscles while participating in Zoom meetings or typing away at my computer.

10. The Bedtime Stretch Routine

Every night before bed, I started a stretching routine. It was my way of telling my body, "Hey, thanks for putting up with my shenanigans today." Stretching helped me wind down, and it also helped with my flexibility. Plus, there's something inherently funny about trying to touch your toes and realizing they're a lot further away than you remembered.

Incorporating these simple, sometimes silly, exercises into my daily routine revolutionized the way I viewed fitness. It wasn't a dreaded task anymore; it was a series of small, fun activities that added up to a healthier, happier me.

I learned that fitness isn't about punishing your body; it's about celebrating it. It's about finding joy in movement, laughter in exertion, and a sense of accomplishment in the smallest of victories. Whether it's carrying heavy grocery bags or laughing your abs into existence, every bit counts. Indeed, one of the trickiest parts of maintaining a fitness routine is finding time in our often hectic schedules. But fear not, for I am here with some crafty hacks to help you squeeze in exercise, even on your busiest days. And yes, I mean it, feel free to put down this book for a bit and give one of these a try. I'll be right here waiting for you when you get back.

1. The Five-Minute Blitz:
  - Believe it or not, even five minutes can make a difference. Choose a high-intensity workout like jumping jacks, push-ups, or squats. Do as many as you can in five minutes. It's a quick way to get your heart rate up and inject some energy into your day.
  - This hack is like finding a shortcut in a game – a quick and effective way to get to your destination, or in this case, your fitness goal.

2. The Commercial Break Workout:
  - Watching TV? Utilize the commercial breaks. Stand up and do a mini-circuit of bodyweight exercises. You could even just march in place. By the end of your show, you'll have racked up a good amount of activity.
  - Think of each commercial break as a mini-challenge or bonus round in your day.

3. The Walk-and-Talk Meetings:
  - If you have a phone call or a casual meeting, take it on the go. Walk while you talk. Not only will it help you get in some steps, but the movement might even spark some creative ideas.
  - It's like adding a mobility feature to your usual static activities, making them more dynamic and productive.

4. The Early Bird Special:

- Consider waking up just 20-30 minutes earlier to get in a quick workout. It's a peaceful time when you're less likely to be interrupted, and it can set a positive tone for the rest of your day.
- It's like getting a head start in a race, giving you an edge over your busy schedule.

5. The Lunchtime Quick-Fit:

- Use part of your lunch break to get in some exercise. A brisk walk, a quick gym session, or even some stretching can be a great way to break up your day and boost your energy levels.
- This strategy is like hitting the refresh button mid-game, recharging you for the afternoon ahead.

6. The Household Task Workout:

- Turn household chores into a workout. Put on some music and add some extra movement to your cleaning routine. Lunges while vacuuming, calf raises while washing dishes, or dancing while dusting can all add up.
- This approach turns mundane tasks into fun and productive workout sessions.

7. The Fitness Buddy System:

- Team up with a friend or family member for regular workout sessions. Not only will this give you a set time to exercise, but it also adds accountability and social fun to your routine.
- Consider this your co-op mode in real life, where teaming up makes the challenge more enjoyable and attainable.

8. The Active Commute:

- If possible, walk or bike to work, or park further away from your destination to add in some extra steps. If you use public transportation, consider getting off a stop early and walking the rest of the way.
- This strategy is like choosing the scenic route in a game, where the journey itself adds value to the overall experience.

Remember, it's not about carving out huge chunks of time; it's about making the most of the time you have. Every bit of movement counts, and these small actions can add up to big results over time. So go ahead, put down this book for a moment and try one of these hacks. I promise I'll be right here, cheering you on, when you get back! So, my dear readers, remember that fitness is a journey, not a destination. It's a journey filled with laughter, creativity, and a whole lot of improvisation. Embrace the odd, the unconventional, and the downright silly. Find what works for you, what makes you smile, and what keeps you moving.

Your fitness story is uniquely yours. Write it with joy, humor, and a healthy dose of self-love. And always remember, the best workout is the one that you actually do – even if it's just laughing at your own jokes.

CHAPTER 4.
YOU ARE WHAT YOU EAT

"You can't outrun a bad diet, but you can certainly try to outwalk it at a brisk pace."

If there's one thing I've learned on this wild ride called 'getting fit,' it's that abs are made in the kitchen. Who knew, right? I always thought they were made in some secret underground lab where they also design those impossible-to-open plastic packages. But as it turns out, what you eat is just as important as your workout routine.

Now, before we dive into the nitty-gritty of healthy eating, let me set the record straight: I am not what you would call a 'foodie.' Unless, of course, you count my uncanny ability to identify the nearest fast-food joint blindfolded. My culinary skills were, let's say, underdeveloped. The microwave was my best friend, and the pizza delivery guy knew me by name.

But as I embarked on this journey to a fitter, healthier me, I knew something had to change. And so, dear readers, I bravely ventured into the unknown territory of... the kitchen.

The Great Kitchen Expedition

Stepping into the kitchen with the intention of cooking something healthy was like setting foot on an alien planet. There were utensils whose names I couldn't pronounce and appliances that looked like they required a pilot's license to operate. But armed with a sense of humor and a slightly overconfident Google search, I began my culinary adventure.

1. The Breakfast Battle

They say breakfast is the most important meal of the day. Well, my breakfast routine used to involve a cup of strong coffee and, on a good day, a stale doughnut. It was time for a change. I started experimenting with oats – and let me tell you, there's more to oats than meets the eye. Overnight oats, oat pancakes, oat muffins – if it could be oated, I tried it. And while not every experiment was a success (oat smoothies are a no-go, trust me), I found that a good breakfast could set the tone for the whole day.

2. The Snack Attack Redux

As a lifelong snacker, the idea of giving up my midday munchies was akin to giving up my firstborn. But instead of reaching for chips or cookies, I started experimenting with healthier options. Hummus became my new best friend. Carrot sticks were no longer just for rabbits. And nuts – who knew there were so many kinds? Almonds, walnuts, cashews – it was like a United Nations of snackable goodness.

3. The Salad Saga

Salads and I had a complicated relationship. I always viewed them as the food equivalent of a participation trophy – nice, but not really what you're after. However, I soon discovered the joy of creating my own salads. Gone were the days of limp lettuce and sad tomatoes. I ventured into the world of arugula, spinach, and kale – vegetables I previously thought were just used as garnishes. I added proteins like grilled chicken, beans, and boiled eggs, and experimented with dressings that didn't come out of a bottle. My salads became a canvas for culinary creativity.

4. The Hydration Station Revolution

Remember when your mom told you to drink more water, and you rolled your eyes? Turns out, Mom was onto something. I used to drink soda like it was the elixir of life. But as I started drinking more water, I noticed a change. I felt better, more energetic, and less like a human raisin. I even started infusing my water with fruits and herbs, turning hydration into a tasty treat.

I continued my quest to stay hydrated, finding new and exciting ways to make water interesting. Herbal teas, both hot and cold, became a staple. I discovered the refreshing taste of cucumber water and the indulgent feel of a splash of fruit juice in sparkling water.

As I journeyed through the world of healthy eating, I learned that it wasn't about strict diets or depriving myself. It was about making better choices, one meal at a time. It was about discovering new flavors and ingredients, and finding joy in the process of nourishing my body.

In the next installment, we'll dive deeper into the kitchen capers, exploring the art of meal prep, the adventure of trying new recipes, and the occasional culinary catastrophe that reminds us all that we're only human.

So, grab your apron (or don't, I rarely do), and let's continue this flavorful journey together. Who knows? You might just find your inner chef, or at least have a good laugh trying.

Having conquered the breakfast battleground and the snack attack with a newfound gusto for greens and grains, it was time to venture further into the uncharted territories of lunch, dinner, and the dreaded realm of desserts.

The Lunchtime Chronicles

Lunch used to be an afterthought for me, often a hasty sandwich or, more often than not, fast food on the go. But as I embraced my new role as a novice nutritionist, lunch became an exciting middle act in my daily food drama.

I discovered the joy of leftovers. Yes, leftovers, the unsung heroes of the lunch world. Cooking a little extra at dinner meant I had a ready-to-go meal for the next day. It was like sending a gift to future me, and future me was always grateful.

I experimented with wraps, salads, and soups, finding that a little creativity could turn even the most mundane ingredients into a midday feast. I learned to appreciate the subtle art of sandwich-making, where whole grain bread, lean meats, and an array of veggies could create a symphony of flavors.

The Dinner Dilemma Decoded

Dinner was where I really started to flex my culinary muscles. Gone were the days of microwavable meals and takeout. I began to see cooking as less of a chore and more of an adventure.

I played with spices, discovering that food didn't have to be drenched in sauce to be flavorful. I learned that herbs were not just decorations but were, in fact, flavor powerhouses. I tried recipes from different cultures, traveling the world from my kitchen, one dish at a time.

Fish, once a mysterious and intimidating ingredient, became a regular on my menu. I learned to bake, broil, and even grill it. Pairing it with a side of steamed vegetables or a colorful salad, I created meals that were not only healthy but also visually appealing. After all, we eat with our eyes first.

The Dessert Dilemma

Ah, desserts, my Achilles heel, my sweet temptation. I've always had a sweet tooth, and the thought of giving up desserts was akin to parting with a dear friend. But instead of a farewell, I opted for a makeover.

I explored the world of healthy desserts. Yes, they exist, and no, they're not all sad substitutes for the real thing. I experimented with fruit-based desserts, like baked apples with cinnamon or poached pears in red wine. I discovered the magic of dark chocolate, a small piece of which could satisfy my chocolate cravings without leading to a sugar-induced coma.

I even dabbled in baking, replacing refined sugars with natural sweeteners like honey or maple syrup, and using whole wheat flour instead of white. My kitchen became a laboratory, where each dessert was a delicious experiment.

The Final Frontier: Meal Prep Mastery

As I became more comfortable in the kitchen, I embraced the concept of meal prep. Spending a few hours on the weekend to prepare meals for the week was not only efficient, but it also ensured that I had healthy options on hand at all times.

I learned to batch cook grains like rice and quinoa, roast a variety of vegetables, and prepare proteins like chicken or tofu. Each meal was a mix-and-match adventure, ensuring variety and preventing boredom.

When I look back at my journey from a fast-food fiend to a home-cooking hero with a sense of pride and a dash of disbelief. I've learned that eating healthy doesn't mean sacrificing flavor or joy. It's about finding balance, experimenting with new foods, and most importantly, enjoying the process. So, to you, fellow adventurers in the world of healthy eating, I say this: be bold, be curious, and always remember that the best ingredient in any dish is a sprinkle of humor and a heaping spoonful of love.

CHAPTER 5.
REMEMBER TO HAVE FUN

"Exercise: because one day, zombies will come, and the couch potatoes will be the first to go." - Yours Truly

It was during a particularly grueling episode of trying (and failing) to touch my toes that I had an epiphany: exercise doesn't have to be about grunts, sweat, and tears. It can be about laughs, creativity, and, dare I say, enjoyment. This groundbreaking revelation led me on a quest to make exercise something I could actually look forward to. A quest that was equal parts comedy and tragedy, with a sprinkle of triumph.

The Quest for Fun Fitness

I began to see my daily routine not as a series of obstacles but as opportunities for spontaneous workouts. Who said you need a gym membership or fancy equipment to Get The F*ck In Shape? Not I, said the guy who once thought a burpee was a polite after-dinner ritual.

1. The Grocery Bag

Grocery shopping – it's something we all have to do, but who knew it could double as a workout? I turned the mundane task of carrying groceries into a strength-building exercise. Each bag was a weight, and every trip from the car to the kitchen was a set. My arms got stronger, and the canned goods stopped feeling like boulders. Plus, it was environmentally friendly – fewer trips meant fewer carbon emissions, right?

2. The Vacuum Tango

House chores are the unsung heroes of the exercise world. Vacuuming, for instance, became a dance. With each push and pull of the vacuum, I added a lunge or a squat. Not only did my floors get cleaner, but my legs also got stronger. And let's be honest, there's something strangely satisfying about turning a boring chore into a mini workout party.

3. The Sofa Stretch

The couch, often seen as the arch-nemesis of fitness, became my stretching buddy. While watching TV, I'd take advantage of commercial breaks to do some stretches. Touching my toes (or attempting to), doing side bends, or simply twisting my torso. It wasn't much, but it was better than sinking further into the couch cushions.

4. The Culinary Cardio

I turned cooking into a cardio session. Chopping vegetables became a race against time. Stirring the pot was a test of endurance. Even waiting for the microwave became an opportunity for calf raises or wall sits. I was no Gordon Ramsay, but I sure could break a sweat dicing onions.

5. The Laughter Workout

Never underestimate the power of laughter as an ab workout. I made it a point to watch or listen to something funny every day, ensuring a good belly laugh. It's said that laughter is the best medicine, and while it might not cure all, it certainly provided a daily dose of abdominal exercise.

Transforming my daily routine into an exercise routine didn't happen overnight. It took trial, error, and a fair amount of self-mockery. But as I discovered, the key to making exercise less dreadful was to stop seeing it as a punishment and start viewing it as a playful, integral part of my day.

So, my fellow fitness travelers, as we journey through this chapter, remember that exercise doesn't have to be a chore. It can be a joy, a laugh, a part of your everyday life. It's about getting creative, finding those little moments to move, and most importantly, not taking yourself too seriously.

As we continue this tale, I'll share more of my adventures in turning the mundane into the muscular, the routine into the remarkable. Stay tuned, and remember: a day without laughter (or a little sweat) is a day wasted.

As I ventured deeper into the jungle of everyday fitness, I discovered that the little things, the quirky routines, were what made exercise not just bearable, but actually kind of fun.

The Whimsical World of Workday Workouts

My day job, like many, involved a lot of sitting. But I found ways to turn even the dullest office day into a fitness opportunity.

6. The Chair Squat Challenge

Who knew that a simple office chair could be the gateway to glute strength? Every hour, on the hour, I performed a series of chair squats. Standing up, sitting down, but never quite letting the chair take all my weight. It was a stealth workout, one that my coworkers never noticed, but my muscles definitely did.

7. The Secret Stairmaster

Taking the stairs instead of the elevator became my daily mini-mountaineering expedition. I challenged myself to take them two at a time, to increase my heart rate and add a bit of zest to my step. Every flight conquered was a small victory, a triumph over the lazy lure of the lift.

8. The Water Cooler Walk

Hydration is key, they say, and I found a way to make it even healthier. Instead of keeping a water bottle at my desk, I walked to the water cooler for each refill. It was a chance to stretch my legs, get my steps in, and catch up on the latest office gossip – a triple win in my book.

Venturing outside, where the air is fresh and the scenery changes, was a revelation. It was exercise disguised as exploration.

9. The Power of the Park

I found a local park and made it my playground. I tried everything from jogging to frisbee, from bird watching (you'd be surprised how much walking it involves) to impromptu yoga sessions on the grass. Each visit was a chance to enjoy nature while giving my body the movement it craved.

10. The Bicycle Diaries

Rediscovering my old bike in the garage was like finding a long-lost friend. I started cycling, initially just around the neighborhood, then gradually venturing further. It was freedom on two wheels. The wind in my hair, the sun on my face, and the satisfying burn in my legs – it was exhilarating.

Bringing my newfound love for movement back home, I explored more ways to stay active within my own four walls.

11. The Cleaning Boogie

House cleaning turned into a dance party. Vacuum to the beat, mop in rhythm, dust with flair. Not only did my house sparkle, but my energy levels soared too. Plus, dancing with a mop is surprisingly therapeutic.

12. The Sofa Balance Beam

While watching TV, I practiced balancing on one foot, then the other, like a gymnast on a balance beam. It was a test of stability and focus, and it usually ended in laughter when I inevitably wobbled too far.

13. The Pillow Fight Workout

And then there was the pillow fight workout. Yes, you read that right. A good old-fashioned pillow fight with my kids (or sometimes, when feeling particularly brave, with my spouse) turned into a whirlwind of activity. It was fun, it was chaotic, and it was a surprisingly effective way to get the heart pumping.

I realized that exercise isn't just about structured workouts or gym routines. It's about finding joy in movement, about turning the ordinary into something extraordinary, and about not taking ourselves too seriously and celebrating every small step and achievement.

In the grand adventure of life, where each day presents its own set of quests and challenges, the art of positive reinforcement is akin to having a loyal sidekick, always ready to remind you of your strengths and victories, no matter how small they may seem. It's about turning the lens through which you view your journey, focusing on progress and positivity rather than disappointment and setbacks.

1. The Victory Dance: Celebrating Small Achievements

- Make it a habit to celebrate your small wins, be it sticking to your workout schedule, choosing a healthy snack, or even getting enough sleep.
- Create your own 'victory dance' or a small ritual to mark these achievements. It could be as simple as a fist pump, a happy dance, or a moment of silent acknowledgment.
- This celebratory act is like earning achievement badges in a game – it validates your efforts and reinforces your motivation to continue.

2. The Positivity Journal: Documenting Your Journey
- Keep a journal or a digital log where you note down your daily or weekly achievements, no matter how small.
- Write down positive experiences, moments of joy, and instances where you overcame a challenge.
- Reviewing this journal is like scrolling through the highlights of your game, reminding you of how far you've come and the battles you've conquered.

3. Reframing Setbacks: Finding the Silver Lining
- Instead of dwelling on disappointments, try to reframe them as learning experiences. Missed a workout? Maybe your body needed rest. Overindulged at dinner? It's a reminder to be more mindful next time.
- This approach is like gaining experience points – every setback teaches you something valuable, making you stronger and wiser for future challenges.

4. Encouraging Self-Talk: Becoming Your Own Cheerleader
- Practice positive self-talk. Counter negative thoughts with affirmations and encouragement. Remind yourself of your strengths and past successes.
- This internal cheerleading is like having an encouraging NPC (non-player character) in your corner, always ready with a word of support and motivation.

5. Sharing Your Progress: Building a Supportive Community
- Share your achievements with friends, family, or a supportive community. Their encouragement and acknowledgment can be powerful motivators.
- This sharing is like joining forces with allies in a game – together, you can celebrate each other's victories and offer support during challenges.

6. Setting Realistic Goals: Achievable Quests

- Set realistic and achievable goals. Instead of lofty, overwhelming targets, break them down into smaller, manageable quests.

- Achieving these smaller goals is like completing side quests – each one brings satisfaction and brings you closer to your ultimate objective.

Incorporating these practices of positive reinforcement into your life is like continuously powering up your character. It helps maintain a sense of enthusiasm and satisfaction on your journey. Remember, every step forward, no matter how small, is progress. Every effort, every choice towards a better you, deserves recognition and celebration. Embrace these moments, for they are the stepping stones to greater achievements. In this game of life, where you are both the player and the creator of your journey, let positivity be your guiding force, turning every challenge into an opportunity and every small step into a victory worth celebrating.

So, my fellow aspiring fitness enthusiasts, as we wrap up this chapter, remember that the journey to fitness is as unique as you are. Find your fun, embrace the quirky, and keep moving, not because you have to, but because it makes you feel good.

Stay tuned for more tales of fitness follies and fun, and remember: life's too short not to enjoy every step, squat, and pillow fight along the way.

CHAPTER 6.
THE MISERY OF MOTIVATION

"The difference between try and triumph is just a little umph!" - Marvin Phillips

The path to fitness is paved with good intentions and the occasional donut detour. My journey was no exception. After embracing the hilarity and humility of starting a fitness routine, the next monumental task was keeping the flame of motivation burning, even when it wanted to sputter and die.

The Dawn of Realization

It dawned on me one morning (and by morning, I mean a barely acceptable hour that should be reserved for sleeping or quietly resenting the chirping of early birds) that motivation wasn't something that just 'happens.' It's something you cultivate, like a bizarre houseplant that needs just the right amount of sunlight, water, and, in my case, desperate pleading.

The Motivational Mixtape

Music became my first line of defense against the siren call of the snooze button. I crafted a playlist so energizing, so invigorating, that it could make a sloth consider a career in aerobics. Each morning, as the first notes played, I'd rise like a phoenix from the ashes of my comforter, ready (or at least more willing) to tackle the day's workout.

The Power of the Fitness Vision Board

I created a vision board, a collage of my fitness goals, inspirational quotes, and pictures of people doing incredible athletic feats that I could barely comprehend, let alone aspire to. This board was a visual pep talk, a daily reminder of where I was heading. It hung on my fridge, turning every trip to grab a snack into a moment of reflection and, sometimes, a change of heart.

The Daily Dose of Humor

I found that laughter was indeed the best medicine, especially when the thought of exercising made me want to curl up and live under my bed. I followed fitness memes, joined online communities, and shared my journey with friends who could laugh along with me. This daily dose of humor kept things in perspective – it's hard to take your struggles too seriously when you're chuckling.

The Great Outdoors as a Motivational Arena

I took my workouts outside whenever I could. Something about the fresh air, the greenery, and the occasional dog happily chasing its tail made exercise feel less like a chore. Whether it was a brisk walk, a gentle jog, or just stretching under the open sky, being outdoors breathed new life into my routine.

The Mini-Goal Method

I set mini-goals, small and achievable milestones that kept me going. It could be something as simple as an extra five minutes on my walk or one more yoga pose. Each mini-goal achieved was a victory, a high-five to myself, and a reason to keep pushing.

The Buddy System in Full Swing

My workout buddy became my fitness co-conspirator. We'd check in on each other, share our triumphs and our less-than-stellar moments. Knowing someone else was in the trenches with me made a world of difference. We celebrated our successes, no matter how small, and commiserated over our shared soreness.

The journey to staying motivated is a rollercoaster of highs and lows, of triumphant fist pumps and moments of wondering if your legs have always been this jelly-like. But the key, I found, is to keep injecting fun, laughter, and a healthy dose of realism into the mix.

In this next part, I'll delve deeper into the strategies that kept me on track, the moments of unexpected inspiration, and the realization that sometimes, it's okay to just do your best and let that be enough.

Continuing my odyssey in the realm of fitness motivation, I delved deeper into the quirky and sometimes absurd methods that kept me tethered to my fitness goals. It was a journey filled with unexpected lessons, laughter, and the occasional motivational hiccup.

Embracing the Fitness Mantra

I discovered the power of a good mantra. It's like having a motivational cheerleader in your head. My mantras ranged from the earnest "You've got this!" to the more whimsical "Don't let the couch win." These little phrases became my mental armor, shielding me from the arrows of laziness and doubt.

The Joy of Rewarding Myself

I learned the art of self-reward. No, not with food – I was trying to be a bit more creative. For every fitness milestone, I'd treat myself to something non-edible but delightful. A new book, a movie night, or that fancy coffee I'd been eyeing. These rewards became beacons of light, guiding me through the darker tunnels of my fitness journey.

The Unexpected Inspiration

Inspiration came from the most unexpected places. A dog determinedly chasing a ball in the park reminded me of the joy in simple, unbridled movement. A child learning to ride a bike, undeterred by falls, reminded me of the power of persistence. Observing the world around me became a source of unexpected motivation.

The Fitness Journal: Tracking the Journey

I started keeping a fitness journal. It wasn't just a log of workouts and meals, but a diary of my journey. I jotted down how I felt, the challenges I faced, and the triumphs, no matter how small. This journal became a testament to my journey, a reminder of how far I'd come, and a motivator to keep going.

The Role of Virtual Challenges

In a world increasingly online, I found virtual fitness challenges. These online communities and apps offered challenges ranging from daily step counts to weekly workout routines. They provided a sense of community and competition that spurred me on, adding an extra layer of accountability and fun.

The Power of Visualization

I practiced visualization. Before each workout, I'd take a moment to close my eyes and envision myself completing the session. I saw myself stronger, fitter, and smiling at the end. This mental imagery set the tone for my workout, filling me with a sense of purpose and possibility.

The Learning Curve

I became a student of fitness. I read articles, watched videos, and listened to podcasts. Learning about fitness made it more interesting and less intimidating. Knowledge became power, power that fueled my motivation.

From mantras to journals, from rewards to virtual challenges, each played a part in keeping me on the path to fitness. So, to you, my fellow journeyers on the path of health and wellness, remember that motivation is a personal recipe. It's a blend of what inspires you, what challenges you, and what brings you joy. Find your mix, embrace your journey, and keep moving forward, one step, one laugh, one triumph at a time.

CHAPTER 7.
SOCIAL HUMILIATION

"If at first you don't succeed, then skydiving definitely isn't for you. Stick to fitness." -
Steven Wright

In the grand theater of fitness, I learned that having an audience could be surprisingly motivating. There's something about knowing that others are watching, cheering, or even just mildly interested in your journey that lights a fire under you. So, I set out to turn my fitness journey into a less solitary endeavor, and let me tell you, it was a ride filled with laughter, support, and the occasional blush-worthy moment.

The Buddy System: My Fitness Lifeline

My journey into the world of shared fitness accountability began with what I like to call the 'Buddy System 2.0.' It wasn't just about having someone to grumble with about sore muscles; it was about building a relationship based on mutual motivation and the occasional gentle ribbing. My workout buddy and I became each other's cheerleaders, therapists, and sometimes, drill sergeants.

We set up a system where missing a workout without a good reason meant facing a 'punishment.' Nothing too harsh – think along the lines of buying coffee for the other for a week or doing the other's least favorite exercise. It was effective, mostly because neither of us liked losing.

The Social Media Gambit

Emboldened by the success of the Buddy System, I decided to up the ante: I turned to social media. I started sharing my fitness journey online – the triumphs, the setbacks, the utterly embarrassing moments (like accidentally locking myself out of my house in running shorts in winter).

The response was overwhelming. Friends, family, even strangers began following my journey, offering words of encouragement, advice, and plenty of good-natured jokes. Each post, each share, became a small pledge of accountability. I was no longer just accountable to myself, but to an entire community that was watching my journey unfold.

The Wonder of Workout Groups

Next, I joined a local workout group. Picture a bunch of people from all walks of life, each with their own fitness goals, but all united by a desire to be healthier (and to complain about burpees). These group workouts turned into weekly highlights. We'd meet at the park, at a local gym, or even someone's backyard, and sweat it out together. The energy was infectious, and the group camaraderie made even the toughest workouts enjoyable.

The Art of Self-Humiliation

I embraced self-humiliation as a form of motivation. I started attending workout classes that were clearly out of my league. There's nothing quite like being the only person in a yoga class who can't touch his toes to keep you humble and motivated. I learned to laugh at myself, to not take my stumbles too seriously, and to appreciate the journey, awkward missteps and all.

The Daily Fitness Routine

I weaved fitness into my daily routine in small but significant ways. Here are a few of the tactics I employed:

- The Walk-and-Talk Meetings: Instead of sitting in a coffee shop, I'd suggest walking meetings. It was amazing how a change of scenery and a bit of movement could spark creativity.
- The Staircase Challenge: I made a rule to always take the stairs. Whether at work, the mall, or even at the airport, I became a stair aficionado.
- The Kitchen Workout: Cooking time became an opportunity for mini-workouts. I'd do squats while waiting for the water to boil or lunges while roasting vegetables in the oven.

My journey into the world of fitness accountability taught me the value of community, the power of sharing, and the importance of not taking myself too seriously. It was a lesson in humility, in pushing my boundaries, and in the joy of shared experiences.

In the next part of this chapter, I'll dive deeper into the tactics that helped me stay on track, the role of technology in my fitness journey, and how embracing the social aspect of fitness turned my journey into an adventure.

The Digital Dimension of Accountability

In the digital age, there's an app for everything, including keeping your fitness aspirations on track. I ventured into the world of fitness apps, where every step, every calorie, and every heartbeat could be monitored, analyzed, and shared.

I found an app that turned walking into a game, where I was running away from virtual zombies. Nothing motivates you to pick up the pace like the sound of the undead on your heels. My daily jogs became less about reluctantly dragging myself around and more about survival in a post-apocalyptic world. It was absurd, it was fun, and it worked.

The Power of Online Communities

I discovered online fitness communities, where people from around the globe shared their fitness journeys, tips, and occasional mishaps. These virtual communities were a source of inspiration and a reminder that I wasn't alone in my struggles. Whether it was a forum, a social media group, or a fitness app community, the encouragement and sense of belonging I found there were invaluable.

Embracing the World of Wearables

I also jumped on the wearable technology bandwagon. My fitness tracker became my constant companion, a tiny digital coach strapped to my wrist. It nudged me to move more, to sleep better, and to compete with friends in friendly step-count competitions. It was like having a personal trainer who was also a bit of a nag, but in the most helpful way.

Tracking the Triumphs and Tribulations

I began to meticulously track my progress, not just in terms of pounds lost or miles run, but in how I felt. My fitness journal evolved into a comprehensive diary where I recorded my workouts, my diet, my moods, and my reflections. This tracking helped me see patterns, understand my body better, and celebrate the small victories that might have otherwise gone unnoticed.

The Surprise Benefits of Accountability

This journey into the world of accountability had some surprising benefits. I found that being accountable to others, whether it was my workout buddy, my social media followers, or my online fitness community, also made me more accountable to myself. It built a sense of integrity and commitment to my fitness goals that went beyond external validation.

Learning to Laugh at Myself

Perhaps the most significant lesson in this journey was learning to laugh at myself. Whether it was a workout fail that I shared online or a funny story about a fitness mishap that I recounted to my workout group, finding humor in the journey made it more enjoyable. It made the tough days easier and the good days even better.

As I conclude this chapter, I realize that the journey to fitness is not just a physical one; it's a social, emotional, and sometimes technological adventure. It's about finding your tribe, embracing the tools at your disposal, and most importantly, enjoying the ride, bumps and all.

To anyone embarking on their own fitness journey, remember that accountability, in whatever form it takes, can be a powerful ally. Find what works for you, embrace the support around you, and never forget to find joy in every step, stretch, and squat.

CHAPTER 8.
REWARDS OF THE VICTORIOUS

"The road to success is dotted with many tempting parking spaces." - Will Rogers

Every journey, especially a fitness journey, is sprinkled with milestones that deserve their moments in the sun. As I navigated my way through the ups and downs of getting fit, I realized that celebrating these moments wasn't just fun; it was crucial. It was a way of acknowledging the hard work, the sweat, and, let's not forget, the occasional tears.

Ballads of Bragging Rights

I became a bard of my own fitness saga, singing (sometimes literally) the tales of my victories. My first successful ten push-ups? That deserved a social media post with a celebratory dance video. The day I finally touched my toes? I called my mom. The first time I jogged a whole mile without stopping? I might have sent a slightly boastful group text to all my friends.

These moments of bragging were not just about puffing up my ego. They were about sharing the joy of achievement. They were my way of saying, "Look what I did, and if I can do it, so can you!"

The Trove of Non-Edible Treasures

I turned my rewards into a treasure hunt. For each goal I reached, I treated myself to something that brought me joy but didn't involve calories. When I lost the first ten pounds, I got myself a new pair of funky workout leggings. After completing my first month of consistent workouts, I splurged on a concert ticket. These rewards were like the loot at the end of a particularly challenging level of a video game.

Celebrating with Creative Flair

I found that the best celebrations were the creative ones. When I achieved my goal of doing yoga every day for a month, I organized a 'Yoga and Yogurt' party. We did a group yoga session in the park, followed by a build-your-own yogurt parfait bar. It was fun, it was different, and it was a celebration that perfectly encapsulated the milestone.

Incorporating Fitness into Daily Life

Fitness became a seamless part of my daily life, almost without me noticing. I'd do calf raises while waiting in line at the grocery store. I'd opt for the bike instead of the car for short trips. I even started doing wall-sits while brushing my teeth. These small actions kept me moving and kept the spirit of fitness alive in my everyday routine.

Reflecting on the Journey

Taking time to reflect on my progress became a ritual. I'd look at old workout logs and marvel at how far I'd come. I'd compare before and after photos, not just to see the physical changes, but to remember the mental and emotional growth that accompanied them.

Sharing the Victories

Sharing my successes became about more than just celebrating; it was about inspiring. I realized that my journey could motivate others. When friends said they started walking more or tried a yoga class because of my posts, it filled me with a sense of purpose that was far greater than any personal milestone.

Your Body is your Temple

Understanding the concept that your body is your temple is crucial for long-term health and wellness. Just like any structure, your body needs a solid foundation, regular maintenance, and care to ensure its longevity and functionality.

1. The Foundation: Building a Strong Base for Health
   - Think of your body's foundation as the basic aspects of health: nutrition, exercise, sleep, and mental well-being. If any of these are compromised, just like a building with a cracked foundation, the entire structure – your body – can be affected.

- Addressing foundational issues such as poor diet, lack of exercise, insufficient sleep, and unmanaged stress is crucial. These are not just the cornerstones of your health; they are the bedrock upon which everything else stands.

2. Regular Maintenance: The Key to Longevity

- Regular maintenance of your body involves consistent habits that promote health. This includes eating a balanced diet, engaging in regular physical activity, getting adequate sleep, and managing stress.
- Just as you wouldn't wait for your car to break down before servicing it, you shouldn't wait for health problems to arise before taking care of your body. Regular 'servicing' of your body keeps it running smoothly and efficiently.

3. Preventive Care: A Proactive Approach

- Preventive care involves taking steps to prevent health problems before they start. This includes regular check-ups and screenings, vaccinations, and being proactive about any signs of trouble.
- It's much like a building undergoing regular inspections to ensure everything is in working order. Catching potential issues early can prevent larger problems down the line.

4. Listening to Your Body: Heeding the Early Warnings

- Your body often gives early warning signs when something is amiss. Ignoring these signs is like ignoring small cracks in a building's walls – eventually, they can lead to significant problems.
- Pay attention to signals such as persistent fatigue, unusual aches and pains, changes in appetite or sleep, and emotional distress. These may be indications that your body needs attention.

5. Mind-Body Connection: Holistic Maintenance

- The mind-body connection is a critical aspect of maintaining your temple. Mental health directly impacts physical health and vice versa. Practices like meditation, mindfulness, and yoga can help maintain this balance.
- Think of these practices as the architectural design of your temple – they not only support the structure but also enhance its beauty and functionality.

6. The Importance of Adaptation: Renovations for Your Body

- Just as buildings need renovations to stay current and functional, your body needs adaptations as you age or as your circumstances change. This could mean adjusting your exercise routine, modifying your diet, or finding new ways to manage stress.
- Adaptation is about evolving your maintenance routine to fit your body's changing needs, ensuring your temple remains strong and resilient.

7. The Role of Self-Care: Regular Upkeep

- Self-care acts like the daily cleaning and upkeep of your temple. This includes taking time for relaxation, engaging in hobbies, connecting with loved ones, and ensuring you have moments of joy and laughter.

- Regular self-care not only maintains your temple but also beautifies it, enhancing your overall quality of life.

In essence, treating your body like a temple is about respect, care, and attention. It's recognizing that prevention and regular maintenance are far more effective and less costly than fixing problems after they occur. By building a strong foundation, performing regular maintenance, practicing preventive care, and adapting to your body's needs, you ensure that your temple – your body – stands strong and majestic for years to come.

I understand that the path to fitness is not just about the exercises and the diet. It's about the celebrations, the shared experiences, and the joy of looking back and realizing how far you've come.

As I journeyed further into the realm of fitness, my appreciation for the small victories and the grand triumphs grew. Each step forward, no matter how small, was a part of a larger tapestry that illustrated my journey from fitness novice to a somewhat more seasoned enthusiast.

Creative Celebrations

My celebrations took on various forms, each reflecting the unique nature of the milestone. When I finally mastered a challenging yoga pose, I treated myself to a professional massage. It was my way of thanking my body for putting up with my demands. This approach to rewards transformed my journey, making each goal feel like an adventure rather than a chore.

The Ripple Effect of Sharing Success

Sharing my fitness victories had an unexpected but delightful ripple effect. Friends and family started to share their own successes and struggles with me, creating a circle of inspiration and support. It was as if my fitness journey had started a wave of motivation that reached far beyond my own expectations.

Fitness Integration in Daily Routines

Integrating fitness into my daily routine became second nature. I found ways to make every task an opportunity to move:

- While cooking, I'd do standing abdominal exercises, like oblique twists.
- During TV time, I replaced the couch with a stability ball, engaging my core while enjoying my favorite shows.
- I made a game of parking farther from store entrances to add a few extra steps to my day.

Reflecting with Gratitude

Reflection became a key part of my routine. I would often look back at where I started and feel a deep sense of gratitude. Not just for the physical changes, but for the mental resilience and emotional growth I experienced. This gratitude turned into a powerful motivator, pushing me to continue on my path.

Continuing the Celebration Beyond Myself

I began to realize that my journey could be a catalyst for others. I started organizing small fitness challenges among friends and family. We'd encourage each other and share our progress. These challenges weren't about competition; they were about building a community of support and celebration.

The Evolution of My Fitness Philosophy

My philosophy on fitness evolved. It was no longer just about losing weight or gaining muscle; it was about living a fuller, healthier life. It was about setting an example for my loved ones and enjoying the journey every step of the way.

Looking Forward with Excitement

As this chapter of my fitness story closes, I look forward to the future with excitement. I know there will be more challenges, more successes, and undoubtedly more humorous mishaps. But I'm ready for them all, armed with a sense of humor, a community of support, and a belief in the power of small victories.

CHAPTER 9.
THE LONG UPHILL ROAD

"Maintenance is key. It's the melody in the symphony of fitness."

The journey of maintaining fitness is a bit like walking a tightrope while juggling flaming torches. It requires balance, focus, and a not-insignificant amount of courage. As I ventured into this phase of my fitness journey, I found that the road to maintenance was lined with both challenges and unexpected delights.

The Daily Ritual of Routine

My first lesson in maintenance was the importance of establishing a routine. Not just any routine, but one that was flexible enough to adapt to life's unpredictabilities. I set up a schedule that accounted for busy days, lazy days, and those rare, mythical days when everything goes according to plan.

Each morning, I greeted the day with a series of stretches that made my body feel less like a creaky door and more like a well-oiled machine. I incorporated a mix of cardio, strength training, and flexibility exercises throughout the week, ensuring that my workouts never felt repetitive or dull.

Variety: The Spice of Fitness Life

The spice that kept my fitness life flavorful was variety. I dabbled in different activities, finding joy in the diversity of movement. One day, I'd be the king of the swimming pool, churning through laps like a human motorboat. The next, I'd be on a hiking trail, communing with nature and tripping over tree roots (gracefully, of course).

I even tried dance classes, where I quickly learned that my sense of rhythm was as questionable as my cooking skills. But the laughter and the sheer joy of moving to music added a new dimension to my workout regimen.

Micro-Goals: Celebrating the Small Wins

In the world of fitness maintenance, I became a micro-goal maestro. These small, achievable goals were my daily victories. Whether it was adding an extra five minutes to my run or mastering a new yoga pose, each micro-goal pushed me forward and kept me engaged.

I celebrated these wins with the enthusiasm of a sports team winning a championship. It could be something as simple as a fist pump or a happy dance in my living room. These celebrations kept the fire of motivation burning bright.

Integrating Movement into Every Day

Integrating fitness into my daily routine became a creative endeavor. I found ways to sneak in exercises throughout my day:

- While brushing my teeth, I'd practice squats or leg raises.
- I'd take the stairs two at a time, transforming every staircase into a personal fitness challenge.
- During phone calls, I'd pace around or even do some discreet lunges.

These small movements added up, turning my entire day into an opportunity for fitness.

Community: My Fitness Fellowship

The community I built around my fitness journey continued to be a source of strength and inspiration. We shared tips, cheered each other on, and sometimes just shared a good laugh over our mutual struggles. This fellowship made the journey less solitary and more joyful.

Sharing the Knowledge

As I grew more confident in my fitness lifestyle, I found joy in sharing what I had learned with others. I became the unofficial fitness advisor among my friends, offering tips, encouragement, and the occasional cautionary tale of overambition.

I realize that it's less about the exercises and more about the mindset. It's about finding joy in movement, embracing the discipline with a smile, and appreciating the journey as much as the destination. In the next part of this chapter, I'll explore more strategies for keeping fitness fresh and engaging, and how embracing the unexpected can lead to some of the most rewarding experiences.

CHAPTER 10.
MAINTAINING MOMENTUM

"In the marathon of life, some play to win but forget that playing is meant to be fun."

As I embarked on the seemingly endless road of maintaining fitness, I discovered that the key to longevity in this journey was not just persistence, but also a good dose of humor and the willingness to adapt.

The Long Haul with Humor

My mantra became, "If you're going to have to do it forever, you might as well make it fun." This mindset turned my fitness routine into a playground rather than a prison. I found joy in the little things: the absurdity of grunting loudly in a quiet gym, the comic sight of struggling to put on a wet swimsuit for swimming laps, or even the slapstick comedy of tripping over a yoga mat.

Creating a Workout Playlist That Doesn't Make You Cry

Music was my constant companion in this journey. But instead of the usual high-energy workout tracks, I started creating playlists with a sense of humor. Songs like "Eye of the Tiger" were followed by "I Will Survive," offering both a beat to move to and a chuckle in between. These playlists lifted my spirits and provided an extra boost of motivation, especially on days when the couch was particularly seductive.

Adapting and Advancing

Change became my new workout buddy. I learned that doing the same routine for too long was like listening to a record on repeat - eventually, it becomes background noise. To keep things fresh, I constantly sought new exercises, new routines, and new ways to challenge myself. I joined different fitness classes, from aerobics to Zumba to kickboxing, reveling in the awkwardness of being a beginner and the thrill of learning something new.

Incorporating Fun into Fitness

I started incorporating elements of play into my workouts. This included things like frisbee in the park, which turned out to be a surprisingly effective way to get in some cardio, or playing tag with my kids, which, aside from being a blast, also counted as interval training.

The 'Gamification' of Exercise

Taking a cue from the world of video games, I 'gamified' my fitness routine. I set up rewards for myself - for every week that I met my workout goals, I'd treat myself to something small but enjoyable, like a movie night or a new book. This system of rewards not only kept me motivated but also made the whole process more enjoyable.

Fitness Challenges with Friends

Nothing quite matches the motivation boost of a little friendly competition. I started organizing monthly fitness challenges with my friends. Who could clock the most steps? Who could swim the most laps? These challenges were less about winning and more about pushing each other to do our best. The bragging rights were just a bonus.

Mindful Movement

I began to focus more on the quality of my movements rather than the quantity. This meant paying attention to my form, understanding the muscles I was working, and connecting with my body on a deeper level. This mindful approach to exercise transformed it from a task into a form of self-care.

This venture into maintaining fitness momentum has been a mix of adaptation, fun, and a little bit of silliness. It's about making each workout an experience, something to look forward to rather than something to get over with.

In the next part of this chapter, I'll delve into more strategies for keeping the fitness journey fresh and engaging, and how embracing a lighthearted approach can lead to a more fulfilling and sustainable fitness lifestyle. The journey of maintaining fitness momentum is much like a rollercoaster ride – it has its highs and lows, unexpected turns, and moments of exhilarating joy. In the latter half of this marathon, I learned that the key to sustaining the fun in fitness lies in continuously finding new ways to challenge and amuse myself.

Reinventing Workouts

Stagnation is the enemy of progress, and in the world of fitness, this meant reinventing my workouts regularly. I became a connoisseur of fitness trends, trying out everything from underwater aerobics to goat yoga (yes, it's a thing). Each new style brought a fresh perspective and, often, a good laugh. I found that when I stopped worrying about looking silly, I opened myself up to a whole new world of fun fitness experiences.

Creating Fitness Adventures

I started planning fitness adventures. These were workouts disguised as exciting escapades. A bike ride to a nearby town, a hike to a beautiful viewpoint, or a day of kayaking – each adventure was a workout in disguise and a new memory in the making.

The Power of Fitness Communities

Engaging with fitness communities, both online and offline, became a staple of my routine. These communities were sources of inspiration, encouragement, and a wealth of knowledge. Sharing stories, tips, and occasional fitness memes made the journey less solitary and more enjoyable. I even started a small fitness blog to document my adventures, which turned into a motivational tool for both myself and my readers.

The Art of Balancing Act

Balance, both literal and figurative, became a central theme in my fitness maintenance. Physically, I incorporated balance exercises into my routine – because there's nothing quite like standing on one leg and trying not to fall over to add a bit of excitement to your day. Figuratively, I learned to balance my workouts with rest, understanding that recovery is just as important as the exercise itself.

Seasonal Variations in Fitness

As the seasons changed, so did my workouts. I embraced outdoor activities in the summer, like swimming and beach volleyball, and in the winter, I turned to indoor rock climbing and yoga. This seasonal variation kept my routine fresh and aligned with the natural rhythm of the year.

Staying Flexible and Open to Change

Flexibility became my motto – and not just in the physical sense. I learned to be flexible with my routine, to listen to my body, and to be open to changing my plan when life threw a curveball. This flexibility helped me stay committed without feeling overwhelmed or rigidly tied to a specific regimen.

Celebrating the Journey

Above all, I celebrated the journey. Each day that I chose to move my body, each healthy choice I made, was a cause for celebration. I learned to appreciate the journey itself, not just the destination. Fitness became more than just a routine; it became a joyful part of my life.

Now that we've got this covered, let's dive into a detailed discussion about how eating habits impact our health, both mentally and physically. Understanding the connection between what we eat and how we feel can be a game-changer in our overall wellness journey.

1. The Building Blocks of Our Body: Nutrition's Role in Physical Health
   - Think of food as the fuel that powers the complex machine that is your body. The quality of this fuel directly impacts how well the machine runs. Nutrient-rich foods like fruits, vegetables, whole grains, lean proteins, and healthy fats are like premium fuel. They provide the essential nutrients needed for energy, muscle repair, immune function, and overall physical health.
   - On the other hand, a diet high in processed foods, sugars, and unhealthy fats is akin to putting subpar fuel into your body. Over time, this can lead to various health issues, such as weight gain, heart disease, and diabetes, much like how a poorly maintained machine starts to break down.

2. The Brain-Gut Connection: How Diet Affects Mental Health

- Our diet also plays a crucial role in our mental health, thanks to the brain-gut connection. The gut is often called the "second brain" because of the many neurotransmitters it produces. A healthy diet promotes a healthy gut microbiome, which in turn positively affects mood and cognitive function.

- Foods rich in omega-3 fatty acids (like salmon and flaxseeds), antioxidants (found in berries and leafy greens), and probiotics (found in yogurt and fermented foods) are particularly beneficial for brain health. They're like the power-ups that boost your mental performance.

- Conversely, diets high in sugar and processed foods can negatively impact mood, exacerbate symptoms of anxiety and depression, and even impair cognitive functions.

3. Energy Levels and Eating Habits

- The type and timing of your meals can significantly influence your energy levels throughout the day. Consistent, balanced meals help maintain steady blood sugar levels, preventing the mid-afternoon slump often experienced after a heavy, carb-laden lunch.

- Incorporating a balance of carbohydrates, proteins, and fats in your meals is like ensuring a steady release of energy, keeping you powered and alert.

4. Sleep Quality and Diet

- What we eat can also affect our sleep. Heavy or rich foods right before bed can lead to discomfort and disrupt sleep, while foods like almonds, turkey, and chamomile tea, which contain nutrients that promote sleep, can help improve sleep quality.

- Think of these sleep-friendly foods as the night-time maintenance crew, helping to ensure your body gets the rest it needs to repair and rejuvenate.

5. The Role of Hydration

- Hydration is another critical aspect of your diet. Water is essential for nearly every bodily function, from aiding digestion to regulating temperature. Dehydration can lead to fatigue, mood swings, and decreased cognitive function.

- Regularly drinking water is like providing the necessary lubrication for the smooth operation of your body's many systems.

6. Mindful Eating: The Connection to Emotional Well-being

- Mindful eating, the practice of being present and aware during meals, can transform your relationship with food. It's about listening to your body's hunger and fullness cues, enjoying the flavors and textures of your food, and appreciating the nourishment it provides.

- This practice can lead to healthier eating habits, improved digestion, and a deeper connection to the experience of eating, contributing to emotional well-being.

In summary, our eating habits play a fundamental role in both our physical and mental health. By choosing nutrient-rich foods, maintaining hydration, practicing mindful eating, and understanding the impact of our diet on our body and mind, we can significantly enhance our overall health and well-being. So next time you sit down for a meal, remember that you're not just eating; you're nourishing your entire being.

The journey of maintaining fitness momentum is a continuous cycle of discovery, challenge, and enjoyment. To anyone on this path, remember to find your own rhythm, embrace new experiences, and most importantly, enjoy the ride. Your fitness journey is your own unique story, filled with its own set of triumphs, challenges, and laughter.

CHAPTER 11.
CONCLUSION: A NEW BEGINNING

"Fitness is like a relationship with yourself. Cheesy pick-up lines and grand gestures don't work here, just consistency and a bit of love."

As I stand (or rather, sit comfortably with a cup of tea) at the end of this whirlwind journey into the world of fitness, I can't help but look back with a mixture of pride, astonishment, and a generous dose of humor. It's been a path paved with sweat, the occasional tear, and many, many laughs.

Reflections and Revelations

When I started this journey, I was like a ship without a rudder in the vast ocean of fitness. I had no direction, no real understanding of what I was doing, and a slightly irrational fear of treadmills. But as I navigated through the choppy waters of workouts, nutrition, and the dreaded burpees, I discovered not just the importance of physical health, but the joy and hilarity that comes with it.

I learned that fitness is not a destination; it's a continuous journey. It's not about achieving a perfect body or mastering every exercise. It's about finding a balance, enjoying the process, and embracing the journey's ups and downs.

The Fit and Funny You

The 'fit and funny me' is someone who can laugh at a failed attempt at a new exercise, who can find joy in a particularly grueling workout, and who understands that a slice of cake won't undo all the hard work. It's someone who looks at fitness not as a chore, but as a delightful part of life.

Integrating Fitness into Everyday Life

I found ways to integrate fitness seamlessly into my daily routine:

- Doing calf raises while brushing my teeth or waiting for the kettle to boil.
- Choosing the stairs over the elevator, turning a mundane decision into a mini-workout.
- Walking or biking for short errands instead of driving.

These small choices added up, making fitness a natural part of my day.

A New Perspective on Health and Happiness

This journey has given me a new perspective on health and happiness. Health isn't just about the physical aspect; it's about mental and emotional well-being. It's about laughing, enjoying life, and finding happiness in the small things – like finally being able to touch your toes or run a mile without feeling like you're about to meet your maker.

The Journey Continues

As I close this book, I know that my fitness journey doesn't end here. It's a new beginning, a continuous path of discovery, growth, and laughter. I look forward to the challenges and triumphs ahead, to the new adventures in fitness and health, and to the countless laughs that await.

To anyone embarking on their fitness journey, remember this: be kind to yourself, find joy in the process, and don't take it too seriously. Your journey is your own, unique and beautiful in its way. Embrace the fit and funny you, and enjoy every step of the way.

CHAPTER 12.
EPILOGUE: THE FUTURE OF FITNESS

"The future is not something we enter. The future is something we create." - Leonard I. Sweet

As I sit here, reflecting on my journey of health and fitness, a journey interspersed with bouts of laughter and occasional muscle aches, I can't help but ponder what the future holds. If there's one thing this adventure has taught me, it's that the path to fitness is as winding and unpredictable as it is rewarding.

Envisioning the Road Ahead

The future of my fitness journey, I imagine, will be much like the past: filled with unexpected turns, new challenges, and a plethora of opportunities to laugh at myself. It's a future where health and humor continue to walk hand in hand, where every stumble is a chance to learn, and every success is a reason to smile.

Integrating Fitness into Life's Journey

The integration of fitness into my daily life will continue to evolve. I see myself trying new activities – perhaps paddleboarding or aerial yoga – always with an open mind and a readiness to laugh at the inevitable bloopers. I envision fitness remaining a joyful pursuit, something I do not out of obligation, but out of love for my body and the endless amusement it provides.

Continued Learning and Exploration

In the future, I plan to continue learning and exploring the vast world of health and fitness. Be it through reading the latest research, experimenting with new nutrition plans, or trying out the latest fitness craze, my journey will be one of continuous discovery and growth.

Sharing the Journey

One of the most rewarding aspects of my fitness journey has been sharing it with others. In the future, I see myself continuing to share my experiences, the good, the bad, and the hilarious, to inspire and encourage others on their paths. Whether it's through writing, speaking, or simply being an example, I hope to contribute to a world where fitness is accessible, enjoyable, and filled with laughter.

The Humor in Fitness

As for humor, it will remain my constant companion on this journey. I will continue to find the funny in my fitness escapades, whether it's a comically failed attempt at a new exercise or the humorous realities of aging gracefully. Laughter, after all, is not just medicine for the soul; it's fuel for the fitness journey.

The Legacy of a Fitness Journey

Looking ahead, I hope to leave a legacy that inspires others to embrace fitness with joy and humor. To show that being fit isn't about being perfect, it's about being persistent, and having a good laugh along the way. It's about creating a future where fitness is a celebration of what our bodies can do and a journey that we look forward to every day.

In the future, I see a world where fitness is not a chore but a choice – a choice to live healthily, laugh often, and enjoy every step of the journey. It's a future that I am excited to create, one workout and one laugh at a time.

So, to anyone reading this, remember that your fitness journey is your own unique story. Embrace it, enjoy it, and don't forget to laugh along the way. The future of fitness is bright, and it's yours to shape.

Final Word: The Cheat Code to Life

If you're going to take away just one gem from the treasure trove of fitness hilarity and wisdom in "Get The F*ck In Shape," let it be this: Stretch. Yes, stretch. Whether you've been running marathons or just marathoning through TV series, stretching is the unsung hero of staying fit with age.

Think of stretching as the cheat code to life. It keeps you limber, reduces the risk of impersonating a robot with each movement, and is key to maintaining your body's version of 'smooth operation.' Imagine reaching for that top shelf or bending to tie your shoes without emitting a sound reminiscent of a creaky door hinge – that's the magic of stretching.

So, if you remember nothing else, remember to stretch. It's a simple, nearly effortless activity that pays off in dividends. Plus, you can totally do it while binge-watching your favorite shows – talk about multitasking!

Stay flexible, friends, in both body and humor. And who knows, with enough stretching, you might just be able to reach for the stars – or at least that bag of chips on the top shelf.

Stretch Your Way to a Healthier You

As we close the curtain on this rollicking adventure of fitness faux pas and triumphant transformations in "Get The F*ck In Shape," let's zero in on one golden nugget of wisdom that's as simple as it is powerful: Stretching. It's the unsung hero of fitness, the quiet achiever in the world of health, and possibly the closest thing we have to a real-life cheat code.

Stretching, my friends, is not just for athletes or yoga enthusiasts. It's for everyone – for you, for me, for the guy who thought a 'downward dog' was a type of hot dog. It's a cornerstone of maintaining flexibility, preventing injury, and keeping your body feeling young, no matter how many candles are on your birthday cake.

So, how do we incorporate this magical element into our daily lives, especially during those moments that don't seem to scream 'workout time'? Here are a few simple, yet effective stretching tips and hacks to sneak them into your everyday routine:

1. The Morning Stretch Ritual:
   Start your day with a full-body stretch. Before you even step out of bed, take a few minutes to stretch your arms overhead, point and flex your feet, and gently twist your torso. It's like sending a friendly memo to your muscles, letting them know the day has begun.

2. The Brush-and-Balance:

While brushing your teeth, stand on one leg to challenge your balance. Switch legs halfway through. Not only does this improve your balance and core strength, but it also adds a bit of fun to a mundane task.

3. The Couch Potato Flex:
Watching TV? Use commercial breaks as a cue to do some seated leg and arm stretches. Reach for your toes, stretch your arms across your body, or do some gentle neck rolls. You'll be giving your body a mini-maintenance session without missing your favorite show.

4. The Desk De-Stressor:
If you're stuck at a desk for long hours, try some simple seated stretches. Shoulder shrugs, wrist rolls, and ankle circles can work wonders. Every hour, stand up and reach for the sky or do a few side bends. It keeps the blood flowing and can help ward off the stiffness that comes from prolonged sitting.

5. The Grocery Line Limber Up:
Stuck in line at the grocery store? Use this time to subtly stretch your calves or do a few discreet torso twists. It's a productive use of waiting time, and you'll be giving your body a little extra care.

6. The Kitchen Counter Calf Raise:
While waiting for the kettle to boil or the microwave to ping, stand at your kitchen counter and do a few calf raises or side stretches. It's a great way to sneak in some stretching while you go about your culinary business.

Remember, stretching is like a gentle love letter to your body – it's a way of saying, "I care about you." It keeps you nimble, reduces the chances of injury, and can even improve your posture. Plus, it's one of the simplest ways to keep your body in tune, especially as you age.

So, as you turn the last pages of this book, take with you the resolve to stretch a little more each day. It's a small habit that can lead to big changes. Stay flexible, both in body and in spirit, and watch as life's little challenges become just a tad easier to navigate. Here's to stretching our way to health, one laugh and one elongated muscle at a time!

Levelling Up: The Game of You vs. You

Welcome to the most entertaining game you'll ever play: becoming the best version of yourself. Think of it as a video game, except the character you're levelling up is you, and the only high score that matters is your own. And the best part? In this game, cheat codes are allowed, especially if they involve chocolate on cheat days.

Your Personal High Score: The Fun of Beating Yesterday's You

Picture this: every day, you get the chance to beat your own high score in the game of life. Did you choose stairs over the elevator? High score! Swapped your latte for a green tea? Ding ding ding, points! Each choice is like racking up points on an arcade game, except you can't put your initials up when you win – unless you write them on your bathroom mirror, which we totally endorse.

Celebrating the Mini-Wins: Because Small Victories are Still Victories

In this game, small victories are a big deal. Managed to drink an extra glass of water? That's like finding a hidden bonus level. Cooked a healthy meal at home instead of ordering in? You just unlocked an achievement. These mini-wins are the secret power-ups in your journey. Celebrate them like you just won a round of your favorite video game.

When the Game Gets Tough: Powering Through Setbacks

Now, just like any good game, there will be challenges and obstacles. Maybe one day you'll hit the snooze button too many times and miss your workout. Or perhaps the siren call of a double-stuffed pizza will be too strong to resist. Guess what? It's not game over. It's just a chance to hit 'continue' and try again. No guilt, no fuss – just a shrug and a chuckle because tomorrow is another opportunity to beat your high score.

Loving the Game: Enjoy Every Level

Here's the key: love the game you're playing. Enjoy every level, every challenge, and every victory. Dance in your living room as if it's the final boss battle. Cook like you're in a gourmet game show. Laugh at your mistakes and cheer on your successes. When you enjoy the process, levelling up doesn't just feel good – it feels great.

Press Play: Your Adventure Awaits

As you close this book and look forward to the rest of your day, remember: you're the hero in the game of your life. You're in competition with yourself, and the prize is feeling fantastic, laughing a lot, and living well. So go ahead, press play, and start chasing those high scores. Here's to you, the soon-to-be champion of your own story, one hilarious, healthy choice at a time.

And now, dear reader, as you flip through these pages and chuckle at my past fitness follies, remember this: feeling good about yourself isn't a level you reach; it's an attitude you carry with you, through the boss battles and bonus rounds of life.

Embrace the Glitches: They're Part of the Game

Your journey will have its glitches – moments when you accidentally eat the whole cake instead of just a slice, or when your yoga pants feel more like a straightjacket. Laugh at these glitches. They're not failures; they're hilarious anecdotes for your autobiography and reminders that perfection is about as real as a unicorn riding a unicycle.

Power-Ups: Find Your Joy in the Little Things

Look for daily power-ups. Maybe it's a song that makes you dance like no one's watching (even though the dog is definitely judging you), or that first sip of coffee that tastes like hope and smells like motivation. These little things are your power-ups, your daily dose of joy that makes you feel good about where you are, right now.

Boss Battles: Celebrate Your Strength

And when you face boss battles – those big challenges like sticking to your workout routine, saying no to the third slice of pizza, or getting through a tough day – celebrate your strength. Whether you come out victorious or in need of a respawn, you're building resilience, character, and a heck of a story to tell.

Multiplayer Mode: Share the Journey

Don't forget to engage in multiplayer mode. Share your journey with friends, family, or anyone who will listen. Celebrate their victories and let them celebrate yours. Laugh together, grow together, and maybe even do a couple of stretches together. Life, like a good game, is better when shared.

Achievement Unlocked: Being Unapologetically You

As you continue on this path, remember, the ultimate achievement is being unapologetically you – a person who finds joy in the ups, learns from the downs, and can laugh at the in-betweens. Keep racking up those experience points by being your awesome self, and remember, in the game of life, you're already winning just by being you.

So there you have it. Keep this guide close, not just as a reminder of how to stay fit, but as a testament to the joy, laughter, and sheer awesomeness of being on this fitness adventure. Keep moving, keep laughing, and most importantly, keep feeling good about yourself, because you, my friend, are doing just great.

As you journey through your day, wielding humor and positivity like a mighty sword, there's one superpower you always have at your disposal – the power of breath. Think of it like a video game hero regaining stamina; each deep breath is a boost to your energy, a recharge to your soul, and a revitalizing force for your body. Here are some simple, yet powerful breathing exercises that can energize you, making you feel like a hero ready to conquer the next challenge:

1. The Power-Up Breath: Deep Belly Breathing
  - Find a comfortable seat or stand with your feet hip-width apart.
  - Place one hand on your chest and the other on your belly.
  - Breathe in deeply through your nose, feeling your belly expand (your chest should move very little).
  - Exhale slowly through your mouth or nose, feeling the belly fall.
  - Repeat this deep belly breathing for 3-5 minutes. Imagine it as filling up your stamina bar, each breath bringing more energy and vitality.

2. The Energizer: The 4-7-8 Technique
  - Inhale quietly through your nose for 4 seconds.
  - Hold your breath for 7 seconds.
  - Exhale completely through your mouth, making a whoosh sound, for 8 seconds.
  - This one breath constitutes a cycle. Repeat this cycle for four breaths.
  - Think of this as a cheat code to calm the mind and energize the body. It's like hitting the refresh button on your internal energy source.

3. The Quick Boost: Kapalabhati (Skull Shining Breath)
  - Sit comfortably with your spine straight.
  - Take a deep breath in.
  - As you exhale, pull your stomach in sharply and quickly, expelling the breath forcefully through your nose. Let your inhalation be passive and natural.
  - Continue this pattern for 15-20 breaths.
  - This rapid breathing technique is like tapping into a quick energy potion. It invigorates the mind, wakes up the body, and fires up your internal engines.

4. The Stamina Saver: Alternate Nostril Breathing
- Sit in a comfortable position with a straight back.
- Place your right thumb over your right nostril and inhale deeply through your left nostril.
- At the peak of inhalation, close off the left nostril with your ring finger, then exhale through the right nostril.
- Continue this pattern, alternating nostrils after each inhalation.
- Spend 3-5 minutes on this exercise. It's like balancing your energy levels, ensuring you're not overloading one side. Think of it as maintaining your health bar in optimal condition.

5. The Relaxing Reset: Sighing Out Loud
- Inhale deeply through your nose.
- Exhale with an audible sigh through your mouth.
- Repeat a few times, letting each sigh release tension and refresh your mind.
- This simple technique is like hitting the reset button, a quick way to release stress and boost your mood.

Remember, in the video game of life, air is your unlimited power source. It's free, it's always available, and it has the incredible ability to rejuvenate your soul and body. So next time you're feeling low on energy, or you need a moment to reset, take a deep breath and imagine yourself powering up, ready to face the world with renewed vigor and vitality. Breath is your secret weapon – use it wisely, and watch as it transforms your everyday challenges into exciting quests and adventures.

APPENDIX A.
THE GET THE F*CK IN SHAPE HALL OF SHAME

Ah, the Hall of Shame – a place where fitness faux pas and workout whoopsies are both celebrated and gently ridiculed. As someone who's had more than my fair share of fitness blunders, I find it only fair to share these tales of caution and hilarity. So, let's dive into some of the most memorable fitness fails and the lessons they offer.

1. The Treadmill Tango

The treadmill: a staple in gyms worldwide and the scene of many a fitness fail. My own misadventure involved stepping onto a treadmill that I didn't realize was already running. The result? A not-so-graceful dance that ended with me sprawled on the floor. The lesson? Always make sure the treadmill is at a complete stop before you embark on your journey to nowhere.

2. The Overzealous Lift

In my early days of strength training, I mistook enthusiasm for expertise. Eager to impress, I loaded up a barbell with more weight than I had ever lifted. The result was a comedy of errors, complete with wobbly knees and a hasty, clattering retreat. The takeaway? Start small, increase gradually, and leave the heroics for superhero movies.

3. The Yoga Faux Pas

Yoga, the art of bending and stretching in ways that look easy until you try them. My most memorable yoga fail involved an attempt at a complicated pose that I had no business trying. Picture a pretzel, but less elegant and more 'help, I can't untangle myself.' The lesson here? Respect your limits and understand that some poses take time (and perhaps a bit of humility) to master.

4. The Aerobics Misstep

Aerobics classes can be a blast, but they can also be a minefield of potential embarrassment. I learned this the hard way when I mistimed a step and ended up colliding with a fellow aerobics enthusiast. It was less of a coordinated dance move and more of an accidental tango. The lesson? Keep an eye on your surroundings and maybe don't position yourself front and center until you've got the hang of the routine.

5. The Swim Sprint Snafu

Swimming: it looks so serene, so graceful. That is until you find yourself gasping for air halfway across the pool because you started your lap like you were racing for Olympic gold. My own overambitious sprint resulted in a very ungraceful doggy paddle to the nearest pool edge. The lesson? Pace yourself, and remember that it's a swimming pool, not a scene from "Jaws."

These tales from the Hall of Shame serve as gentle reminders that in the world of fitness, blunders are part of the journey. They teach us, humble us, and most importantly, give us something to laugh about. So embrace your fitness fails, learn from them, and keep moving forward – with a smile.

APPENDIX B.
THE LAZY PERSON'S GUIDE TO FITNESS

Welcome to the Lazy Person's Guide to Fitness Terms, where we take the jargon of the fitness world and translate it into plain, (mostly) unexaggerated English. Because let's face it, sometimes fitness terms sound like they come from another planet.

1. Aerobic Exercise
- Usual Definition: Any form of exercise that uses oxygen to meet energy demands during exercise through aerobic metabolism.
- Lazy Definition: Exercise that makes you breathe hard enough to blow out birthday candles. Think jogging, cycling, or power-walking away from responsibilities.

2. Anaerobic Exercise
- Usual Definition: Physical exercise intense enough to cause lactate formation, generally short-lasting, high-intensity activity.
- Lazy Definition: The kind of workout that makes you wish you'd never left your couch. It's like aerobic exercise but feels like you're running from a bear.

3. Reps
- Usual Definition: Short for repetitions, it refers to the number of times you perform a specific exercise.
- Lazy Definition: How many times you lift something before wondering why you're voluntarily torturing yourself.

4. Sets
- Usual Definition: A group of repetitions performed without resting.
- Lazy Definition: The number of times you repeat those reps before you start bargaining with the universe for strength.

5. High-Intensity Interval Training (HIIT)
- Usual Definition: A form of interval training, a cardiovascular exercise strategy alternating short periods of intense anaerobic exercise with less intense recovery periods.
- Lazy Definition: A workout routine that tricks you into exercising hard for a short time by promising a rest right after. Spoiler: It's still hard.

6. Plyometrics
- Usual Definition: Exercises in which muscles exert maximum force in short intervals to increase power.
- Lazy Definition: Jump around. Jump up, jump up and get down. It's like being a human kangaroo but less fun.

7. Cardio
- Usual Definition: Cardiovascular exercise designed to increase heart rate and improve oxygen consumption.
- Lazy Definition: Any exercise that makes you question your life choices as you gasp for breath. Often involves running to nowhere on a treadmill.

8. Core
- Usual Definition: Refers to the muscles in your pelvis, lower back, hips, and abdomen.
- Lazy Definition: The mythical area of your body you're supposed to work out to get abs. Also, a great place to balance snacks.

9. Yoga
- Usual Definition: A group of physical, mental, and spiritual practices that originated in ancient India.
- Lazy Definition: Stretching and bending in ways that make you realize how un-flexible you really are, often followed by a nap (known as savasana).

10. Cool Down
- Usual Definition: A period of low-impact or slower exercise following a more intense workout.
- Lazy Definition: The glorious time when you realize the workout is almost over and you're still alive.

This guide to fitness terms is designed to bring a smile to your face and a little bit of clarity to the sometimes-baffling world of fitness jargon. Remember, fitness can be fun, and understanding it doesn't have to be a workout in itself!

APPENDIX C.
REST UP HERO

Let's explore the profound impact of sleeping habits on both our physical and mental health. Sleep, often underrated, is actually a cornerstone of overall wellness, much like the foundation of a building – essential for keeping everything stable and functioning.

1. Physical Health and Sleep: The Regeneration Period
- During sleep, our bodies undergo critical repair and regeneration processes. This is the time when muscle growth, tissue repair, and protein synthesis primarily occur. Poor sleep can hinder these processes, leading to slower recovery from exercise, reduced muscle growth, and an overall decrease in physical performance.
- Sleep also plays a vital role in maintaining a healthy immune system. Lack of sleep can weaken immune function, making you more susceptible to infections and illnesses. It's like leaving the fortress gates open for invaders.

2. Weight Management and Sleep: The Hormonal Balance
- Sleep significantly impacts two critical hunger hormones: ghrelin (which stimulates appetite) and leptin (which signals fullness). Lack of sleep can increase ghrelin levels and decrease leptin, leading to increased hunger and appetite, often resulting in weight gain.
- Additionally, when you're sleep-deprived, the body craves high-fat, high-carbohydrate foods for quick energy. It's like your body going into emergency mode, seeking the fastest fuel source to compensate for the lack of rest.

3. Mental Health and Sleep: The Mind's Restoration
- Quality sleep is crucial for cognitive functions such as memory, learning, decision-making, and problem-solving. During sleep, the brain consolidates memories and clears out toxins. Poor sleep can lead to decreased concentration, impaired cognitive function, and, in the long term, increased risk of neurological disorders.

- Lack of sleep is also closely linked to mental health issues such as depression, anxiety, and mood swings. It's as if the brain's emotional processing center becomes less effective, making it harder to cope with stress and maintain emotional stability.

4. Sleep and Heart Health: The Silent Guardian
- Adequate sleep is essential for heart health. Chronic sleep deprivation has been linked to an increased risk of heart disease, high blood pressure, and stroke. During sleep, heart rate and blood pressure naturally lower, giving your heart a much-needed rest.

5. The Sleep-Creativity Connection: The Dream State
- REM sleep, in particular, seems to play a significant role in creativity and problem-solving. It's during this phase of sleep that the brain can make new and innovative connections between ideas – it's like your brain is brainstorming without the confines of conscious thought.

6. Sleep Hygiene: Practices for Better Sleep
- Establishing a regular sleep schedule helps regulate your body's internal clock. Going to bed and waking up at the same time every day (even on weekends) can significantly improve the quality of your sleep.
- Creating a bedtime ritual, like reading or meditating, signals to your body that it's time to wind down. Avoiding screens and bright lights before bed can also help as they can disrupt the production of melatonin, the hormone responsible for sleepiness.
- Ensuring your sleep environment is conducive to rest is also crucial. This includes a comfortable mattress, a cool room temperature, and minimal noise and light.

7. Napping: The Mini Reset
- Short naps, around 20-30 minutes, can be beneficial, especially for those who have trouble getting enough sleep at night. They can improve mood, alertness, and performance. However, longer naps or napping late in the day can interfere with nighttime sleep.

In essence, sleep is not just a passive state of rest; it's an active period of restoration for both the mind and body. By prioritizing good sleep habits, you're investing in your physical health, mental clarity, emotional stability, and overall quality of life. So, consider your time asleep as essential as the time you spend awake – it's a crucial component of your health and well-being journey.

APPENDIX D.
THE PARADIGM SHIFT _____

1. Enhanced Physical Health:
- The most obvious impact is on physical health. A more active lifestyle can lead to weight loss, improved cardiovascular health, stronger muscles, and better overall fitness. It's like upgrading your body's operating system – everything just works better.

2. Improved Mental Health:
- Exercise isn't just good for the body; it's a boon for the mind as well. Regular physical activity can lead to reductions in symptoms of anxiety and depression. It's like clearing the cache in your brain – everything becomes a bit more streamlined and efficient.

3. Boost in Energy Levels:
- As counterintuitive as it may seem, being more active actually increases your energy levels. It's like unlocking a hidden energy reserve you never knew you had. You'll find yourself more equipped to handle daily tasks with vitality and enthusiasm.

4. Better Sleep:
- Regular physical activity can help regulate your sleep patterns. Think of it as fine-tuning your internal clock. Better sleep leads to more alertness during the day and an overall healthier lifestyle.

5. Enhanced Cognitive Function:
- Exercise has been shown to boost brain function. It's akin to adding extra RAM to your mental processes. You might find yourself thinking more clearly, learning more quickly, and improving your memory.

6. Increased Confidence and Self-Esteem:
- As you meet your fitness goals and improve your physical health, you'll likely experience a boost in self-confidence and self-esteem. It's like levelling up in a game – with each achievement, you feel more powerful and capable.

7. Improved Relationships:
- This new lifestyle can positively impact your relationships. Whether it's through shared activities or simply being in a better mood more often, you'll likely find improvements in how you interact with others.

8. Better Stress Management:
- Physical activity is an effective stress reliever. It's like having a built-in pressure release valve, helping you manage stress in a healthy and productive way.

9. Longevity and Quality of Life:
- An active lifestyle can contribute to a longer life and, just as importantly, a better quality of life during those years. It's like ensuring that the game of life doesn't just last longer, but also gets more enjoyable and fulfilling.

10. A More Positive Outlook:
- Last but not least, the shift to an active lifestyle often brings a more positive outlook on life. It's like switching from a black-and-white view to full color – everything seems more vibrant and hopeful.

In essence, changing your paradigm to embrace health and fitness can be transformative. It's about more than just the physical benefits; it's a holistic upgrade to your quality of life. This new lifestyle becomes a canvas on which you paint a more vibrant, energized, and fulfilled life. So embrace the change, and watch as every facet of your life starts to reflect this new, dynamic you!

APPENDIX E.
THE MIND-BODY CONNECTION

In the epic quest of health and fitness, while we often focus on the physical aspect, the power of the mind is like a hidden treasure waiting to be discovered. Mindfulness is your secret tool in this adventure, akin to acquiring a mystical artifact that enhances your abilities. It's about being present, aware, and fully engaged in the moment. Here are some simple mindfulness exercises that can help fortify your mental health, creating a solid foundation for your physical well-being:

1. The Mindful Minute: A Quick Mental Reset
- Find a quiet place to sit or stand comfortably.
- Set a timer for one minute.
- During this minute, focus entirely on your breathing. Notice the sensation of the air entering and leaving your body.
- If your mind wanders (and it will), gently guide it back to your breath.
- This exercise, although brief, is like hitting the pause button in a hectic game, giving you a moment of calm amidst the chaos.

2. The Sensory Explorer: Engaging Your Five Senses
- Take a moment to engage each of your five senses one by one.
- Focus on five things you can see around you. It could be the color of the sky, the pattern on a fabric, anything.
- Then, concentrate on four things you can touch. Feel the texture of different objects or the air on your skin.
- Notice three things you can hear, even subtle sounds like the distant hum of traffic or the rustling of leaves.
- Identify two things you can smell. Maybe it's the aroma of coffee or the scent of a flower.
- Lastly, focus on one thing you can taste, even if it's just the lingering flavor of your last meal or drink.
- This exercise is like equipping your character with enhanced sensory perception, heightening your awareness and grounding you in the present.

3. The Mindful Walk: A Journey of Awareness
- Go for a walk, preferably in a natural setting, but anywhere will do.
- As you walk, pay close attention to the sensation of your feet touching the ground.
- Observe your surroundings with intention, noticing things you might usually overlook.
- This mindful walk is like a side quest in your day, an opportunity to connect with your environment and find peace in the simple act of walking.

4. The Gratitude Log: Counting Your Blessings
- Take a few minutes each day to write down three things you're grateful for.
- They can be as significant as a personal achievement or as simple as a delicious meal.
- This exercise is akin to collecting valuable items on a quest – each note of gratitude adds to your mental wealth and enhances your overall well-being.

5. The Body Scan: Tuning into Your Physical Self
- Lie down in a comfortable position.
- Starting from the top of your head, gradually bring your attention to different parts of your body.
- Notice any sensations, tension, or discomfort. Don't judge or try to change these sensations; just observe them.
- This body scan is like conducting a status check on your character, ensuring each part is in optimal condition for the adventures ahead.

Incorporating these mindfulness exercises into your daily routine is like equipping your character with armor and tools necessary for the challenges ahead. A healthy mind not only supports a healthy body but also enhances your overall experience of life's journey. By being mindful, you're not just going through the motions; you're actively participating in and enjoying each moment. It's a journey of discovery, where you learn to appreciate the now, reduce stress, and cultivate a sense of inner peace that radiates through all aspects of your health and life.

ABOUT THE AUTHOR.
INDIANA JETHRO BUMSTEAD

My journey from a fitness-phobic to a fitness fanatic is a tale filled with humor, unexpected twists, and a healthy dose of self-deprecation. Growing up, my idea of a workout was reaching for the remote control and occasionally lifting a slice of pizza to my mouth. I viewed gym-goers with a mix of awe and suspicion, wondering why anyone would subject themselves to such torture voluntarily. My fitness journey began not with a thunderous epiphany but with a quiet, nagging realization that perhaps being winded by a flight of stairs wasn't a badge of honour. The first time I set foot in a gym, I felt like an alien landing on a new planet. I gawked at the machines, puzzled by their purpose and mechanics. It was a world both intimidating and fascinating.

As I stumbled through my early days of working out, I quickly became a connoisseur of gym bloopers. From flying off a treadmill like a misguided missile to mistaking a gym regular for a personal trainer (and asking him for help), my misadventures were both humbling and, in retrospect, hilarious. Gradually, something miraculous happened. I started to enjoy exercising. The feeling of accomplishment after a workout, the camaraderie with fellow gym-goers, and the newfound energy I felt began to outweigh the initial discomfort. I discovered the joy of movement, the thrill of pushing my limits, and the satisfaction of setting and achieving goals. As my fitness journey progressed, I transformed not just physically, but mentally and emotionally. I learned that fitness was less about having six-pack abs and more about feeling strong, healthy, and confident. I became a fitness fanatic, not because I loved the gym, but because I loved how it made me feel.

Throughout my journey, humor has been my constant companion. I learned to laugh at my mistakes, to find the humor in challenging situations, and to not take myself too seriously. This philosophy of humor and health is what I aim to share through my writing, hoping to inspire others to embark on their own fitness journeys. So, there you have it: the story of Indiana Jethro Bumstead, a man who went from dodging exercise to embracing it with open arms (and a few good laughs). My journey is a testament to the fact that fitness can be fun, fulfilling, and occasionally funny. Whether you're a fitness phobic or a fanatic, remember that the journey is as important as the destination, and a little laughter along the way makes everything better.

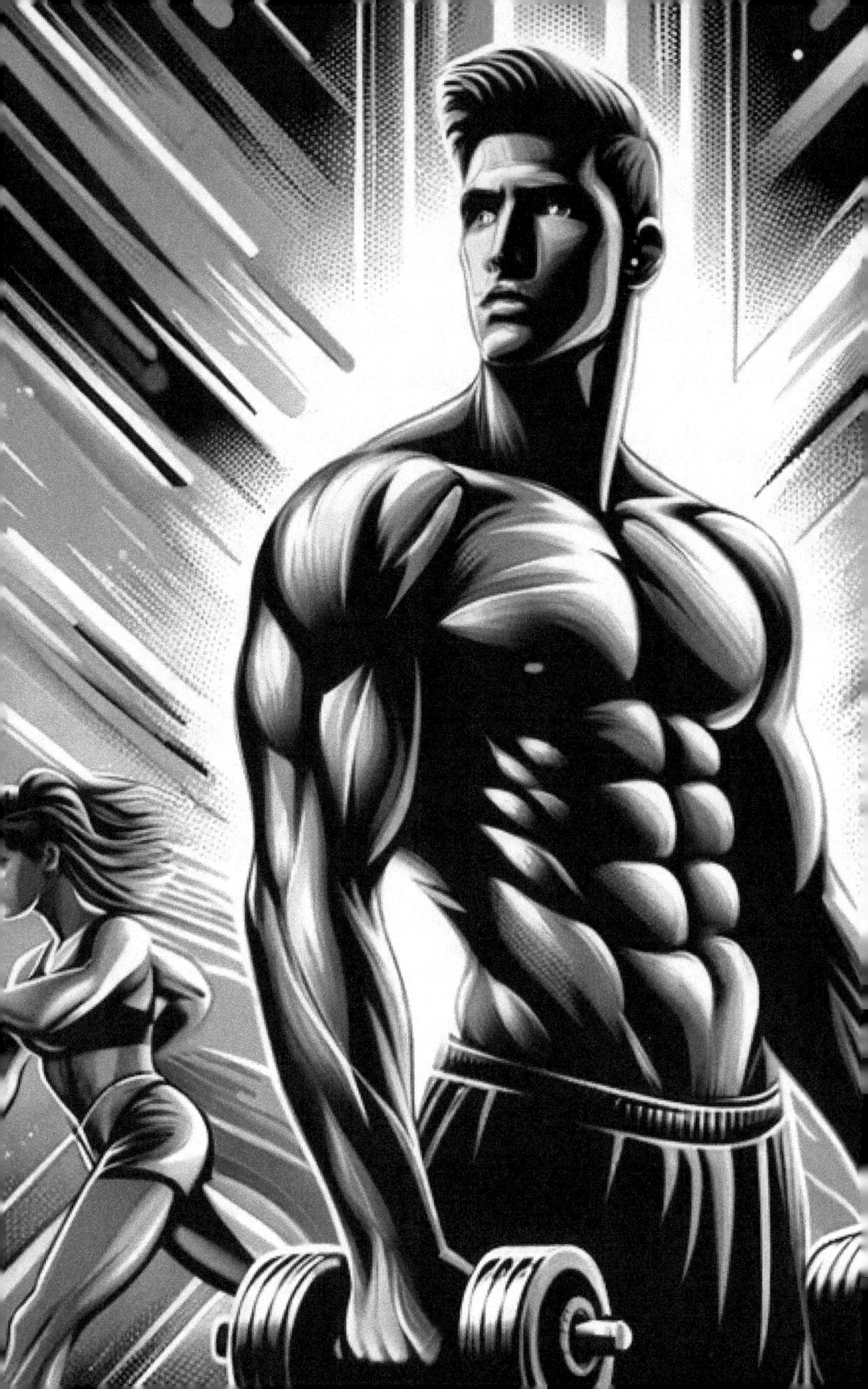

LEGAL DISCLAIMER

This book, titled "Get The F*ck In Shape : A Guide for the Fitnessly-Challenged" by Indiana Jethro Bumstead, is intended for entertainment and motivational purposes only. The content provided herein does not constitute professional medical, nutritional, or physical therapy advice or instructions.

The author, Indiana Jethro Bumstead, and the publisher, Extra-Extra Publishing, are not healthcare professionals. The information and stories shared within these pages are based on the author's personal experiences and should not be taken as professional guidance.

The reader should understand that participating in any exercise program can result in physical injury. The exercises and advice described in this book are not suitable for everyone, and readers should consult with a physician or qualified health professional before beginning any new exercise, nutrition, or wellness program, especially if they have a pre-existing health condition or concern.

Indiana Jethro Bumstead and Extra-Extra Publishing disclaim any liability from injury or damage that may result from the use of any information, exercises, or suggestions contained in this book. The reader assumes all risks associated with any and all activities and exercises described in this book.

The narratives and anecdotes in this book are provided to entertain and inspire and should not replace the advice and guidance of medical, nutritional, or fitness professionals. Always train, stretch, and exercise responsibly, and seek the advice and supervision of professionals when appropriate.

By reading this book, you acknowledge and agree that neither the author nor the publisher is responsible for accidents, injuries, or health complications that may result from practicing or attempting any of the activities or advice described in this book. Any action you take upon the information in this book is strictly at your own risk.

-

First Edition - December 2023.
Extra-Extra Publishing Company
ISBN: 978-1-7382357-3-5